END EMOTIONAL OVEREATING *NOW*

A Breakthrough Program to Take Control Over Food and Your Life

Daniel G. Amen, M.D.
Larry Momaya, M.D.

MindWorks Press
A Division of Amen Clinics, Inc.

MEDICAL DISCLAIMER

The information presented in this book is the result of years of practice experience and clinical research by the author. The information in this book, by necessity, is of a general nature and not a substitute for an evaluation or treatment by a competent medical specialist. If you believe you are in need of medical interventions please see a medical practitioner as soon as possible. The stories in this book are true. The names and circumstances of the stories have been changed to protect the anonymity of patients.

Copyright © 2011 by Daniel G. Amen, M.D. and Larry Momaya, M.D.

All rights reserved. No part of this publication may be reproduced, stored in a retrieval system, or transmitted in any form or by any means, electronic, mechanical, photocopying, recording, or otherwise, without written permission of the publisher.

Published in the United States by MindWorks Press,
A division of Amen Clinics, Inc., California.
www.amenclinics.com

ISBN: 978-1-886554-33-7

Printed in the United States of America

Other Books By Dr. Amen

The Amen Solution

Unchain Your Brain

Wired for Success

Change Your Brain, Change Your Body, New York Times Bestseller

Magnificent Mind at Any Age, New York Times Bestseller

Sex on the Brain

Making a Good Brain Great, Amazon Book of the Year

What I Learned from a Penguin: A Story on How to Help People Change

Preventing Alzheimer's

Healing Anxiety and Depression

New Skills for Frazzled Parents

Healing the Hardware of the Soul

Images of Human Behavior: A Brain SPECT Atlas

Healing ADD

How to Get out of Your Own Way

Change Your Brain, Change Your Life, New York Times Bestseller

ADD in Intimate Relationships

Would You Give 2 Minutes a Day for a Lifetime of Love

A Teenager's Guide to ADD

Mindcoach: Teaching Kids to Think Positive and Feel Good

Ten Steps to Building Values Within Children

The Secrets of Successful Students

TABLE OF CONTENTS

INTRODUCTION ... 7

Chapter 1: UNDERSTANDING YOUR RELATIONSHIP WITH FOOD ... 12
Breaking Up Doesn't Have to Be Hard to Do

Chapter 2: KNOW YOUR NUMBERS AND BOOST YOUR BRAIN ... 20
Optimize Your Brain's Hardware to Improve Your Emotional Health

Chapter 3: KNOW YOUR VALUES AND MOTIVATORS ... 35
What's Driving Your Desire to Get Healthy?

Chapter 4: CORRECT NEGATIVE THOUGHTS ... 51
Change Your Thinking to Change Your Eating Habits

Chapter 5: MANAGE YOUR STRESS ... 76
Meditation and Deep-Breathing Exercises to Calm Stress

Chapter 6: EAT MORE MINDFULLY ... 84
Meditate on Your Meals Rather Than Munching Mindlessly

Chapter 7: LIKE TO DISLIKE ... 90
Yes, You Can Stop Craving the Foods You Overeat

Chapter 8: DISCONNECT THE BRIDGES FROM THE PAST ... 101
Learn From the Past Without Emotionally Reliving It

Chapter 9: TAME YOUR INNER CHILD ... 115
Learn to Say "No" to Yourself and Others

Chapter 10: EMERGENCY RESCUE FOR SETBACKS ... 129
Tips to Help You Stay on Track

ACKNOWLEDGMENTS ... 138

INTRODUCTION

When you feel stressed or upset, do you turn to food as a way to soothe your emotions? I've certainly done that. I remember one day when I dealt with four suicidal patients, two violent teenagers, and two couples who hated each other. When I got home I felt like I deserved all seven of the chocolate chip cookies I ate.

As children we were loved, soothed, bribed, celebrated, and rewarded with food. We cry and the easiest way to get us to stop is to give us a lollipop or a cookie. We win the T-ball game and are rewarded by going out for pizza. We're told that if we behave in church we'll get a doughnut for being good. We celebrate our birthdays with cake and ice cream.

On each of these occasions, an intricate network of brain systems and neurotransmitters is hard at work encoding these experiences. Each time, your brain lays down neural tracks connecting its reward center, the part of the brain that makes you feel pleasure, to its memory centers. Over time, these nerve cell connections become strengthened and eventually they become so embedded within your brain that they become habits, essentially unconscious responses.

   Feel bad → eat a cookie → feel better

   Do something good → eat pizza → feel great

   Need an incentive → dangle a doughnut as a reward → finish your project and get that reward

   Want to celebrate → indulge in cake and ice cream → feel special

It's no wonder so many of us turn to food when we feel stressed, frustrated, mad, sad, fearful, anxious, or even happy. For many of us, emotional eating has been encoded in our brains since we were small children.

For others of us, the encoding is tied to a traumatic event or series of events, such as physical or emotional abuse, an accident, or witnessing a disaster. During times of heightened stress, the brain's memory centers shift into overdrive and the events, the emotions, and the way you ate to soothe yourself become etched into your unconscious. This can create a pattern of emotional overeating that you will feel compelled to repeat over and over again.

That's part of why losing weight can be so hard. Your conscious mind knows what you need to do to lose weight—eat right and exercise, for example—but your unconscious mind fights back. It resists rewriting that code that has been laid down over years and years. Your conscious mind rationally tells you, "Don't eat the cheesecake because it is loaded with fat, calories, and sugar that will make me gain weight." But your unconscious mind urges you to replay your habitual scenario, "Go ahead and eat the cheesecake because it will make you feel better."

The wrestling match between your conscious mind and unconscious mind sets you up for a lifetime of yo-yo dieting—being good for a few days, weeks, or months then falling back into the old comfortable patterns that are making you fat and unhappy. To get off the emotional overeating rollercoaster, you have to address this struggle inside your brain.

What if I told you that you could get your unconscious mind to stop fighting you and start helping you instead?

You can!

Recruit Your Unconscious Mind to Help You End Emotional Overeating NOW

At Amen Clinics, Inc. we have been using brain imaging for the past two decades to help us see what is going on inside our patients' brains. Brain imaging has proven to be such a valuable tool in helping us diagnose and treat our patients that I always say, "How do you know unless you look?"

With emotional overeating, there's an additional component, and as my co-author and colleague, Larry Momaya, M.D., likes to say, "How do you know unless you look into the unconscious mind?"

Larry and I have both seen mind-body techniques play an important role in helping people change their eating behaviors so they can lose weight and get the body they have always wanted. That's why we have created this groundbreaking program that helps you harness the power of your own unconscious mind to help you put an end to emotional overeating.

Before I tell you about the program, let me introduce you to Larry, who is one of the most popular and highest-rated psychiatrists in the Amen Clinics Newport Beach office. Larry specializes in some very powerful techniques that work with the unconscious mind, including some life-changing techniques that you may not be familiar with. Using these techniques, he has helped numerous patients break free from the foods they crave, whether it's chocolate, bagels, coffee, ice cream, or cheeseburgers. Take Derek, for example.

[To make this program easier to read and to avoid the confusion that can arise when two authors are co-writing a book, we decided to write it in my voice and then have passages from Larry where he details the unique set of therapeutic tools he uses to help his patients end emotional overeating NOW. We have put these passages, like the following, in italics.]

Derek had absolutely no control over his desire to eat chocolate. For example, he would be driving down the freeway, and all of a sudden, he would get such an intense urge for chocolate that he would have to pull off the freeway, stop at a gas station, buy a chocolate bar, and eat it right there on the side of the road.

Desperate to kick his craving for chocolate, Derek came to see me. Using one of the techniques you will learn about in this program, I guided Derek to replace all the wonderful qualities he loved so much about chocolate with the thing he hated most—celery.

At the end of our very first session, I presented Derek with some gourmet chocolate and asked him if he had any desire to eat it.

> *Derek said, "No."*
>
> *I put the chocolate in Derek's hand and asked, "What do you feel like doing?"*
>
> *"Nothing."*
>
> *"Do you feel like eating this?"*
>
> *"No."*
>
> *"What do you want to do with it?"*
>
> *"Throw it out."*

Amazingly, Derek hasn't eaten any chocolate since that day. ***And he doesn't miss it at all!***

This last part is one of the things, which makes this program so completely different from any other emotional overeating plan. Most plans tell you to avoid the foods you crave and the situations and people that encourage you to overeat. But when you use these techniques involving the unconscious mind, you no longer have to avoid the foods, people, or places that fuel your overeating. You are free.

*For example, Derek can have his favorite chocolate bar in his hands and have absolutely **no** desire to eat it. This is the end of fighting with yourself and the ultimate freedom from the foods you crave.*

Derek's experience is just one example of the many ways your unconscious mind can be the answer to ending emotional overeating.

The End Emotional Overeating NOW Program

In this program, you will discover a variety of tools that can help you recruit your unconscious mind to end emotional overeating NOW. You will learn:

- Why you have such a strong relationship with some foods and how to get out of a "bad relationship"

- What you can do to boost your brain so you are better able to rewire it

- What's really driving you to change your habits

- Tools to correct the negative thoughts that sabotage your efforts

- Strategies to calm the stress that sends you running to the refrigerator

- Tips to help you become more aware of what you're eating and why

- How a powerful technique can help you say goodbye to the negative emotions that have been fueling your eating problems

- How a certain technique can help you stop eating the foods you crave

- How to prevent other people, places, and things from triggering your emotional overeating

- Ways to make sure you stay on track even when things get tough

Larry and I know that the practical and powerful tools in this program work. We have seen it transform the eating habits of our patients at Amen Clinics and know that it can help you end emotional overeating NOW.

Let's get started.

Chapter 1

UNDERSTANDING YOUR RELATIONSHIP WITH FOOD

Breaking Up Doesn't Have to Be Hard to Do

I've had my share of relationships. Some of them have been wonderful relationships that put a pep in my step and made me feel like I was on top of the world. But some of them have been bad relationships that made me look and feel awful.

I'm talking about my relationships with food.

There was Diet Coke®. For a certain period of my life, I felt like it was my best friend. It perked me up for a while, but eventually let me down. And the aspartame gave me pain in my joints that made me feel like an old man.

There was fudge. Sweet, sweet fudge. Eating a piece of fudge could instantly transport me back to my childhood, conjuring up happy memories of me standing at the stove making fudge with my grandfather who was a candy maker and my best friend. Whenever I felt nervous, frustrated, or sad, eating fudge could take me back to those happy times and make me feel better. Plus, I thought I was honoring my grandfather's memory by eating fudge. But as a neuroscientist and psychiatrist, I knew that the sugar, fat, and salt were working on the heroin centers of my brain and giving me brain fog, in addition to making me gain weight.

Then there was Rocky Road ice cream. The chocolate-y richness, crunchy almonds, and those cute little marshmallows were always there for me at the end of a long day. I would eat it at night as a way to reward myself for a hard day's work and to help me unwind. We spent many nights together, but I always felt guilty about our trysts because I knew it was contributing to the extra 25 pounds I was carrying around.

I knew I had to break up with all of these foods.

I traded in Diet Coke® for green tea and almost instantly felt more energetic and eliminated the joint pain.

Breaking up with fudge was really hard for me because it felt like I was breaking up with my grandfather. Indulging in fudge was what I did to feel close to him long after he had passed away. I had to find another way to feel that closeness to him without the fudge.

As for the Rocky Road ice cream, I tried giving it the boot several times but I kept letting it creep back into my life. It had become an automatic habit like I talked about in the Introduction. If it was nighttime, I *needed* my bowl of Rocky Road. When I finally admitted to myself that I was stuck in a bad relationship and couldn't get out, I went to Larry for help. Using one of the techniques in this program, Larry helped me recruit my unconscious mind to say goodbye to Rocky Road ice cream for good.

With my unconscious mind on board, breaking up was so easy to do. It can be for you, too. But first you need to 'fess up to your food relationships.

Are You Having A Relationship With Your Food?

If you're reading this, I'll bet you are. Relationships with food can take many forms. Becoming aware of the kind of relationship you have with food, what it means to you, and why you can't get out of it is very important.

Food affairs can be very similar to personal relationships. For example:
- When you feel blue you may turn to one friend who always makes you laugh.

- When you feel anxious you may reach out to your parents who calm your nerves.

- When you feel angry you may head straight to your next-door neighbor to vent.

- When you want to reminisce about the good ol' days you may call a childhood friend.

- When you want to feel loved you may seek out the opposite sex.

If you're like a lot of people, food may be the "friend" you turn to in order to help you cope with any or *all* of these emotional needs. When these emotions start to bubble up, it makes you feel uncomfortable, and you use food to stuff them back inside you so you won't have to deal with them.

And unlike friends, neighbors, lovers, or even spouses who may eventually go their separate ways, your favorite food will stick by you through thick and thin. You can always count on that pizza, cheeseburger, or soda to be there for you to fill that emotional need just like it has every other time before.

It's just like being stuck in a bad personal relationship. You probably know people, perhaps yourself included, who stay in a rotten relationship even though they know it's no good for them and even though all their friends keep advising them to get out of it.

Why do people do that? Some prefer *any* relationship, even a bad one, to no relationship at all. Some find comfort in the familiar, no matter how bad, and are so afraid of the unknown that it keeps them coming back for more.

It's the same thing with food. You know on a conscious level that the cheesecake, doughnuts, or chips are harming your health, making you fat, and making you feel worse about yourself. People around you, like your doctor, your mother, or your best friend, are urging you to just say "no" to the foods that are making you miserable. But you just can't kick them out of your life. That's why Larry says,

When you are not working as a team with your own unconscious mind, breaking up with food can be so hard to do.

Take Janine, 26, for example. She came to see me because she wanted to break up with Cheez-Its®. Janine had been diagnosed with a gluten sensitivity, so she knew that eating the cheesy snack crackers wasn't doing her brain or body any favors. But she couldn't resist.

When I worked with her on giving up the snack, Janine started feeling very sad. I asked her why, and she said, "Because eating Cheez-Its® reminds me of coming home from school and eating them with my friends. Those were really happy times for me, and I'm afraid I'm going to miss that now."

*I worked with Janine on those thoughts and helped her unconscious mind discover that her memories of her friends were **not** neatly encased in little cheesy snack crackers sold in store aisles. Her memories resided within her, and she could access them anytime she wanted. When her unconscious mind recognized this, it was no longer a struggle to give up the Cheez-Its®.*

My Food Relationships
Write down the foods you have relationships with and the type of relationship you have with it (fear, anger, sadness, guilt, happy, etc.)

Food   **Type of Relationship**

_____   _____

_____   _____

_____   _____

Is Your Relationship With Food Defining Who You Are?

Rita, 67, had been drinking one to two cans of Pepsi ™ soda every single day without fail for 55 years! Talk about a long-term relationship! She loved the soft drink so much, the people in her office called her "the Pepsi lady." And she thought of herself as "the Pepsi lady." But she had no idea that every time someone called her that or she called herself that, it reinforced the grip that Pepsi ™ had on her unconscious mind.

*That's because the words you use to **describe** yourself ultimately **define** yourself.*

The more people call you "the Pepsi lady" or "the pizza guy" or "the dessert queen" and the more you call yourself those names, the more you begin to associate with it. It's suggestion from the outside and auto-suggestion, which is remarkably similar to the way hypnosis works on the unconscious mind. The unconscious mind hears the suggestion and then follows the suggestion and plays it out.

*If you're "the pizza guy" and someone offers you a slice of pepperoni pizza, well **of course** you're going to take it. After all, you're "the pizza guy," right?*

Be very careful with the words you use to describe yourself. The first step to getting away from such "name-calling" is recognizing the words you use to describe and define yourself.

My Food-Related Identity
Write down any ways you describe yourself that involve food.

_____

_____

_____

_____

_____

_____

Do You Need to Break Up With Yourself?

When you identify yourself with a food, breaking up with it can feel like you're losing your own identity. Rita wondered, "If I'm not 'the Pepsi lady' anymore, who will I be?" This funnels down to very fundamental questions about who we are, how we see ourselves, and how others see us.

You probably thought that emotional overeating was only affecting your waistline. But it affects so much more than that. I'll bet you had no idea just how much your relationships with food were impacting who you are and how you live your life.

Leaving behind your image of yourself is typically one of the hardest things to do and one of the biggest reasons why people remain enslaved to emotional overeating. But it doesn't have to be that hard. With your unconscious mind on your side, it becomes much easier to shift your perception of yourself.

It worked for Rita. After 55 years of identifying herself with Pepsi ™, she quit drinking it and completely lost her desire for it after just one session *with me. In a follow-up session, I asked her how she felt about ending her relationship with Pepsi ™ and she told him, "Before, Pepsi was my friend, and now I can be my own friend. I'm a precious human being, and I deserve to take care of myself."*

What an amazing, life-changing transformation!

At first, it was difficult for Rita's co-workers to come to terms with the "new" Pepsi-less Rita. But when they saw how easily she had transitioned away from her former habit, they became intrigued. Several of them asked Rita how she did it and admitted that they wanted help overcoming their own emotional eating issues.

When you change the way you view yourself, you help others believe that they can change their own self-images, too. In addition, this shift in perception can help you do far more than just lose weight. It can also make you more likely to go for the things you really want in life, ultimately making you more successful and happier. [Incidentally, when you change the way you view yourself, you also end up changing the way you view others, your 'projections'.]

For me, when I stopped being the "fudge doctor" and the "Rocky Road doctor," it led to a change in the way I view myself, which in turn, sparked a number of other changes that helped me lose 25 pounds and feel better than ever.

I am convinced that if my grandfather were alive today, and he knew what the fudge had been doing to my brain health, my weight, and my emotional health, he would be very happy that I had ended my relationship with it. Now I honor his memory by *not* eating fudge.

Who is the Real Me?
Write down positive ways to describe yourself that do not involve food.

_____

_____

Chapter 2

KNOW YOUR NUMBERS AND BOOST YOUR BRAIN

Optimize Your Brain's Hardware to Improve Your Emotional Health

If your brain isn't working right, it will be very hard to overcome emotional overeating. Think of your brain as the supercomputer that runs your life. Like a computer, it has both hardware and software. If there's a problem with your computer's hardware, nothing works right. It's the same with your brain's hardware. When something's wrong, it makes it very difficult to fight emotional eating or follow a healthy eating program, regardless of how amazing it is.

In terms of software, think of your conscious mind as the programs you open and work in on a daily basis, like word processing or spreadsheets on your computer. For example, the 10 steps to brain healthy eating you can find in *The Amen Solution* and the strategies in *Change Your Brain, Change Your Body* are programs your conscious mind puts into action.

Your unconscious mind is more like your computer's operating system, which runs in the background without you having to open it or start it. It's on all the time even though you aren't aware of it. Glitches here can cause computer software programs to crash and can prevent you from following through on the practical solutions you know you should be following.

In this chapter, we will focus on your brain's hardware. When it comes to the health of your brain's hardware, there are some numbers that are critical to know. When these numbers are out of whack, it can keep you enslaved to emotional overeating.

Optimizing these numbers can be one of the keys to helping you get off the emotional rollercoaster so you can achieve your weight loss goals and feel better. You can track your important numbers in our interactive online *Daily Journal* at www.amenclinics.com.

Know your Body Mass Index (BMI). This number tells you the health of your weight compared to your height. To calculate your BMI, use the BMI calculator at www.amenclinics.com. Here's what the numbers mean.

> Underweight: below 18.5
> Healthy: 18.5 – 24.9
> Overweight: 25 – 29.9
> Obese: 30 – 39.9
> Morbidly obese: 40 or over

Knowing your BMI is important for a number of reasons. First, being overweight negatively affects brain function. Dr. Raji Cyrus and colleagues from the University of Pittsburgh found that *people who were overweight, who had a BMI between 25 and 30, had 4 percent less brain tissue and their brains looked eight years older than healthy-weight people! People who were obese, who had a BMI over 30, had 8 percent less brain tissue, and their brains looked 16 years older than healthy-weight people!*

At Amen Clinics, we refer to this as the "dinosaur syndrome." What's that, you ask? Big body… little brain… become extinct.

Knowing your BMI also stops you from lying to yourself about your weight. I [Daniel] was sitting at dinner recently with a friend who seemed totally indifferent about his weight, even though he was injecting himself with insulin for his diabetes at the table. As we were talking, I calculated his BMI for him. Trust me, I can be a very irritating friend if I think you are not taking care of yourself. His BMI was just over 30, in the obese range. That really got his attention, and since then he has lost 20 pounds and is more committed to getting healthy. The truth will set you free. Know your BMI.

Know your Waist to Height Ratio (WHtR). Another way to measure the health of your weight is called your waist to height ratio. Some researchers believe this number is even more accurate than your BMI. BMI does not take into account an individual's frame, gender, or the amount of muscle mass versus fat mass. For example, two people can have the same BMI, even if one is much more muscular and carrying far less abdominal fat than the other; this is because BMI does not account for differences in fat distribution.

The WHtR is thought to give a more accurate assessment of health since the most dangerous place to carry weight is in the abdomen. Fat in the abdomen, which is associated with a larger waist, is metabolically active and triggers the brain to produce various hormones that can cause harmful effects, such as diabetes, elevated blood pressure, and altered lipid (blood fat) levels.

Many athletes, both male and female, who often have a higher percentage of muscle and a lower percentage of body fat, have relatively high BMIs but their WHtRs are within a healthy range. This also holds true for women who have a "pear" rather than an "apple" shape.

The WHtR is calculated by dividing waist size by height, and takes gender into account. As an example, a male with a 32-inch waist who is 5'10" (70 inches) would divide 32 by 70, to get a WHtR of 45.7 percent. The following chart helps you determine if your WHtR falls in a healthy range (these ratios are percentages):

Women
- Ratio less than 35: Abnormally Slim to Underweight
- Ratio 35 to 42: Extremely Slim
- Ratio 42 to 49: Healthy
- Ratio 49 to 54: Overweight
- Ratio 54 to 58: Seriously Overweight
- Ratio over 58: Highly Obese

Men
- Ratio less than 35: Abnormally Slim to Underweight
- Ratio 35 to 43: Extremely slim

- Ratio 43 to 53: Healthy
- Ratio 53 to 58: Overweight
- Ratio 58 to 63: Extremely Overweight/Obese
- Ratio over 63: Highly Obese

Know your calorie counts. You need to know how many calories you need to eat a day to maintain your current weight, how many calories to eat to lose weight, and how many calories you are actually eating. You can find calorie counters at www.amenclinics.com. Regularly eating more calories than you need not only gives you love handles, but also causes an imbalance in the brain's self-control circuit. It reduces activity in the prefrontal cortex, the brain's brake. This is the area of the brain that tells you to say "no" to the cupcakes. At the same time, it increases activity in the emotional memory centers of the brain, which makes the cupcakes even more desirable to you. When the self-control circuit is out of balance, the cupcakes will always win.

Know the number of hours you sleep at night. Don't fool yourself into thinking you only need a few hours of sleep. Getting less than seven hours of sleep at night is associated with lower overall blood flow to the brain, which leads to more cravings, more bad decisions, and more fat on your body. Strive to get seven or, even better, eight hours of sleep every night. Teenagers need to get at least nine hours a night.

Know the number of fruits and vegetables a day you eat. Count them! Eat more vegetables than fruits and try to get that number to between five and 10 servings to enhance your brain and lower your risk for cancer. A lack of nutrients lowers overall brain function.

Get screening laboratory tests and your blood pressure tested to optimize your brain and body. Here are tests we order at Amen Clinics for our weight-loss groups. When your numbers on these tests are off, it can affect the way your brain's hardware functions. Ask your health care provider to order these tests as part of a healthy brain/body program.

Complete Blood Count—to check the health of your blood. People with low blood count can feel anxious and tired, and may overeat as a way to medicate themselves. People with alcohol problems may have large red blood cells.

General metabolic panel—to check the health of your liver, kidneys, fasting blood sugar, and cholesterol.

Vitamin D level—Low levels of vitamin D have been associated with obesity, depression, cognitive impairment, heart disease, reduced immunity, cancer, psychosis, and all causes of mortality. Have your physician check your 25-hydroxy vitamin D level, and if it is low get more sunshine and/or take a vitamin D3 supplement. I [Daniel] have to take 10,000 international units of Vitamin D3 a day to keep my levels near high normal. Here's what the results mean:

> Low < 30
> Optimal 50 – 90
> High > 100

Thyroid—An overactive thyroid can mimic symptoms of anxiety that make you want to eat as a way to calm down. Having low thyroid levels decreases overall brain activity, which can impair your thinking, judgment, and self-control, and make it very hard for you to lose weight. Have your doctor check your free T3 and TSH levels to check for hypothyroidism or hyperthyroidism and treat as necessary to normalize.

C-reactive protein—This is a measure of inflammation that your doctor can check with a simple blood test. Elevated inflammation is associated with a number of diseases and conditions and should prompt you to eliminate bad brain habits and get thin. Fats cells produce chemicals called cytokines that increase inflammation in your body.

HgA1C—This test shows your average blood sugar levels over the past two to three months and is used to diagnose diabetes and prediabetes. Normal results for a nondiabetic person are in the range of 4 to 5.6 percent. Prediabetes is indicated by levels in the 5.7 to 6.4 percent range. Numbers higher than that may indicate diabetes. Diabetes narrows the arteries, making the brain more susceptible to tiny strokes and gradual damage. Diabetes is also associated with a decline in cognitive function.

DHEA and free and total serum testosterone level—Low levels of the hormones DHEA and testosterone, for men or women, have been associated with low energy, cardiovascular disease, obesity, low libido, depression, and Alzheimer's disease.

Blood pressure—Have your doctor check your blood pressure at your yearly physical or more often if it is high. High blood pressure is associated with lower overall brain function, which means more bad decisions.

Know how many of the 12 most important modifiable health risk factors you have, then work to decrease them. Here is a list from researchers at the Harvard School of Public Health. *Check the ones that apply to you.*

- ☐ Smoking—constricts blood flow to the brain
- ☐ High blood pressure—lowers overall brain function
- ☐ BMI indicating overweight or obese—as your weight goes up, the physical size of your brain goes down
- ☐ Physical inactivity—lowers blood flow to the brain
- ☐ High fasting blood glucose—associated with prediabetes, diabetes, and insulin resistance, which has been linked to inflammation and dementia
- ☐ High LDL cholesterol—associated with late-onset Alzheimer's disease
- ☐ Alcohol abuse—impairs brain function
- ☐ Low omega-3 fatty acids—seen in people with depression, ADD, dementia
- ☐ High dietary saturated fat intake—impairs concentration and memory
- ☐ Low polyunsaturated fat intake—depletes DHA in the brain

- ☐ High dietary salt—contributes to high blood pressure
- ☐ Low intake of fruits and vegetables—lack of nutrients lowers brain function

MY IMPORTANT NUMBERS

Keep track of your numbers here or use the interactive tools on our website.

BMI _____
WHtR _____
Calorie counts
    Calories needed to maintain current weight _____
    Calories needed to lose 1 pound per week _____
    Calories I actually consume each day _____
Number of hours I sleep _____
Number of fruits and veggies I eat per day _____
CBC _____
Metabolic panel _____
Vitamin D _____
Thyroid _____
C-reactive protein _____
HgA1c _____
DHEA and testosterone _____
Blood pressure _____
Number of modifiable health risks I have _____

Boost Your Brain

Your brain is involved in everything you do, including how you think, how you feel, how you act, and even how you eat. When your brain works right, you work right, and when your brain is troubled you are much more likely to have trouble in your life. With a healthy brain you are happier, wealthier, wiser, and you just make better decisions; when your brain is not healthy, for whatever reason, you are sadder, poorer, less wise and less effective.

One of the most important steps to ending emotional overeating is boosting the actual physical functioning of your brain. When your brain's hardware is functioning at its best, it helps keep your emotions under control so you don't feel compelled to eat in order to soothe yourself.

So how do you get a better brain? Here are tips everyone should follow.

Avoid things that hurt your brain:

- Brain injuries—even mild trauma can cause major problems with your brain's hardware

- Drug and alcohol abuse—cause imbalances in the brain's reward system and impair brain function, plus drinking every day is associated with having a smaller brain

- Chronic stress—tells your brain to release hormones that increase your appetite and cravings

- Smoking—constricts blood flow

- Too much caffeine—restricts blood flow to the brain

- Too much TV—associated with ADD in children and Alzheimer's disease in adults, and increases your risk for obesity

- Dehydration—even mild dehydration lowers brain function, drink half your weight in ounces every day

- Lack of exercise—lowers blood flow

- Negative thinking—lowers brain activity

- Excessive texting and social networking on the Internet—associated with attention problems

Engage regularly in brain healthy habits:

- Protect your brain

- Eat a highly nutritious diet

- Get adequate sleep

- Exercise

- Learn something new every day—keeps your mind sharp

- Use relaxation techniques to cope with stress—improves mood, reduces blood pressure, and calms your brain

- Practice gratitude—when you focus on what you love, your brain works better

- Take some simple supplements, like a multivitamin and fish oil

- Treat mental disorders—mental disorders are brain disorders, treating them enhances brain function

My Bad Brain Habits	**My Brain Healthy Habits**
Write down the daily habits you have that harm your brain	*Write down the daily habits you have that help your brain*
_____	_____
_____	_____
_____	_____
_____	_____
_____	_____

If you would like some help remembering to practice brain healthy habits, you can find daily reminders on our website.

Know Your Brain Type

To fully optimize your brain, it is a good idea to know your brain type. Based on our brain imaging work at Amen Clinics, we have identified five types of overeaters based on brain patterns. We have seen patterns associated with brains that tended to be compulsive, some were impulsive, others were sad, and still others anxious, in various combinations. This is exactly the reason why most diets don't work. They take a one-size-fits-all approach, which based on our brain imaging work, makes absolutely no sense at all.

Knowing your individual brain type is critical to balancing your brain so you can end emotional overeating. Be aware that each of the five types can be associated with emotional overeating. You can take a test on our website to find your brain type. Here is a brief summary of each type.

Brain Type 1: "The Compulsive Overeater"

People with this type tend to get stuck on the thought of food and feel compulsively driven to eat. They often say that they have no control over food and tend to be nighttime eaters because they worry and have trouble sleeping.

Compulsive overeaters generally have too much activity in the front part of their brains, usually due to low levels of a chemical called serotonin, so they overfocus and can get stuck on the same thought, such as the ice cream in the freezer that is calling their name. They can also get stuck on negative thoughts that make them feel bad, which makes them use food to deal with those feelings.

Caffeine and diet pills usually make people with this type anxious, because their brains do not need more stimulation, and they often feel as though they need a glass of wine at night, or two or three, to calm their worries.

Compulsive overeaters do best when we find natural ways to increase serotonin. Serotonin is calming to the brain. Physical exercise boosts serotonin as does using certain supplements, such as 5-HTP, saffron, inositol, L-tryptophan or St. John's Wort. 5-HTP actually has good scientific evidence that it can be helpful for weight loss, and in my experience, I have found it to be especially helpful for this type.

Brain Type 1 Action Plan

- Eat complex carbohydrates
- Exercise—routine is often helpful
- Avoid nighttime eating
- Learn to distract yourself when you get stuck on thoughts
- Have options
- Avoid automatically opposing others
- Supplements: 5-HTP, saffron, inositol, L-tryptophan, St. John's Wort

Brain Type 2: "The Impulsive Overeater"

People with this type have poor impulse control, get distracted easily, and just reach for food mindlessly. Their brain scans show low activity in the front part of the brain in an area called the prefrontal cortex.

Think of the prefrontal cortex like the brain's brake. It stops you from saying stupid things or making bad decisions. It is the little voice in your head that helps you decide between the banana and the banana split.

When you're an emotional overeater, having poor impulse control can lead to binges that expand your waistline and leave you feeling bad about yourself.

Impulsive overeating is common among people who have attention deficit disorder (ADD), which has been associated with low dopamine levels in the brain. People with ADD often struggle with a short attention span, distractibility, disorganization, and impulsivity. Research suggests that having untreated ADD nearly doubles the risk for being overweight. And, without proper treatment, it is nearly impossible for these people to be consistent with any nutrition plan. Overweight smokers and heavy coffee drinkers also tend to fit this type.

We help impulsive overeaters by boosting dopamine levels in the brain and strengthening the prefrontal cortex. Higher-protein, lower-carbohydrate diets tend to help, as does exercise and certain stimulating medications or supplements, such as green tea, rhodiola, or L-tyrosine. Any supplement or medicine that calms the brain, such as 5-HTP, typically makes this type *worse* because it can lower both your worries and your impulse control.

Brain Type 2 Action Plan

- Eat a higher-protein diet that's lower in simple carbohydrates
- Exercise at least 30 minutes every day
- Set goals (see the One-Page Miracle exercise in Chapter 3)
- Enlist someone you trust to provide outside supervision for you
- Avoid impulsively saying "yes"
- Supplements: green tea, rhodiola, L-tyrosine

Brain Type 3: "The Impulsive-Compulsive Overeater" (a combination of types 1 and 2)

On the surface, it seems almost contradictory. How can you be both impulsive and compulsive at the same time? Think of compulsive gamblers. These are people who are compulsively driven to gamble and yet have very little control over their impulses. It is often the same with emotional overeaters.

Our scans tend to show too much activity in the brain's gear shifter, so people over think and get stuck on negative thoughts, but they also have too little activity in the prefrontal cortex so they have trouble supervising their own behavior.

Emotional overeaters with this type benefit from treatments that increase both serotonin and dopamine, such as exercise with a combination of supplements like 5-HTP and green tea.

Brain Type 3 Action Plan

- Eat a balanced brain healthy diet
- Exercise at least 30 minutes every day
- Set goals (see the One-Page Miracle exercise in Chapter 3)
- Avoid automatically saying "no"
- Avoid impulsively saying "yes"
- Have options
- Distract yourself if you get stuck on thoughts
- Supplements: combine green tea and 5-HTP

Brain Type 4: "The Sad or Emotional Overeater"

People with this type overeat to medicate their feelings of sadness and to calm the emotional storms in their brains. They often struggle with depression, low energy, low self-esteem, and pain symptoms, and they tend to gain weight in winter. Their brain scans tend to show too much activity in the limbic or emotional part of the brain.

For this type, exercise, fish oil, optimizing vitamin D levels, and certain supplements, such as SAMe, can be very helpful to balance the brain, improve your mood, help with energy, and decrease pain.

Brain Type 4 Action Plan

- Exercise at least 30 minutes 4-5 times a week
- Correct negative thoughts
- Write down five things you are grateful for every day
- Volunteer to help others
- Work to strengthen your relationships
- Supplements: fish oil, vitamin D, DHEA, SAMe; for sleep: melatonin

Brain Type 5: "The Anxious Overeater"

People with this type medicate their feelings of anxiety or nervousness with food. They often complain of waiting for something bad to happen and frequently suffer from headaches and stomach problems.

Their brain scans often show too much activity in an area called the basal ganglia. This part of the brain is involved in setting a person's anxiety level. When there is too much activity here, due to low levels of a chemical called GABA, people often have anxiety and physical tension.

The best treatment for this type is to soothe the brain with meditation, prayer, and deep-breathing exercises, plus using a combination of B6, magnesium, and GABA.

Brain Type 5 Action Plan

- Exercise at least 30 minutes 4-5 times a week
- Try relaxation techniques: meditation, prayer, deep-breathing exercises
- Correct negative thoughts
- Supplements: GABA, vitamin B6, magnesium, lemon balm; for sleep, kava kava or valerian root

You can find out much more about brain types on our website. After you take the brain type test on our website, write your brain type here along with your brain type action plan.

My Brain Type

_____

My Brain Type Action Plan

_____

_____

_____

_____

_____

_____

Keep Track of Your Emotions

To end emotional overeating, you must be aware of the things that trigger your emotions. Keep a daily journal to help you track your emotions and eating habits. On a daily basis, rate your moods, anxiety, and stress levels, and write down everything you eat. Also keep track of your sleep, exercise, thinking patterns, and energy levels.

By keeping a journal, you will begin to notice patterns, which is an important step to changing your habits. After working with thousands of patients, I have discovered that this can help keep you motivated and improve your success. You can find an interactive daily journal on our website.

Chapter 3

KNOW YOUR VALUES AND MOTIVATORS

What's Driving Your Desire to Get Healthy?

Why do you care about ending emotional overeating and getting healthy? It is such a basic question, but if you don't understand what is truly driving your desire to change, then your chances of success are diminished. It is critical to get in touch with the reasons why you want to get healthy. Here, Larry describes how he helps patients do that.

When doing Values work with people who are emotional overeaters, I ask them what is important to them about being healthy. Let's do a quick exercise. Spend some time thinking about why you want to end emotional overeating and write down 5-10 or them here.

Why I Want to Get Healthy

_____

_____

_____

_____

_____

_____

_____

Now leave this list alone for a while and meet Charlie. When Charlie came to see me, he weighed 350 pounds and had a serious love-hate relationship with butter. He wanted to say goodbye to his emotional overeating and had read about this program in Amen Clinics' weekly Brain in the News *email newsletter. But Charlie was skeptical, as many people are.*

At the end of our first session, he wasn't skeptical anymore. I went to the office kitchen, found a stick of butter, put it on a paper towel, and brought it back to my office where I offered it to him. Charlie turned his head away in disgust. "Hey, that really worked!" he exclaimed. "I have no desire to eat that." Charlie hasn't eaten butter or anything containing butter *since that day many months ago.*

But Charlie's transformation wasn't finished. Yes, he had given up the butter, but we needed to work on what was driving Charlie's desire to overcome his emotional eating. During one 90-minute session, I elicited what was important to Charlie about his health. In other words, what were his values, and what were the motivators underlying these values. He came up with a list of sixteen things, including:

> *"I want to reverse my diabetes."*
>
> *"I don't want to be out of control anymore."*
>
> *"I don't want anything bad to happen to my wife."*

What do you notice about each of these phrases? They all contain negative *motivators. The problem with negative motivators is that they are* not *helping you get what you want. They are getting you* away from *what you* don't *want. There's a big difference. Allow me to explain:*

Let's say your main value is like Charlie's: "I want to reverse my diabetes." On the surface, that sounds like a good goal. But what happens after you have changed your ways and your diabetes is reversed or under control? Your goal no longer applies. So the main motivating factor for you to end your emotional overeating is gone. What happens next? You start overeating again.

I have seen this happen many times. It's the classic blueprint for yo-yo dieters like Charlie, who had been losing weight and gaining it back for most of his adult life.

To be fair, sometimes a negative motivator can be useful in the short-term to light a fire under you to change your ways. In fact, a recent physicians survey found that sudden events impacting health was by far the #1 factor motivating patients to initiate lifestyle changes to overcome obesity. But it's the motivators that get you moving toward *what you want that are going to keep you motivated in the long run.*

If positive motivators are best, some of you may be wondering why we chose to call this book End Emotional Overeating NOW, *which is technically an 'away from' motivator. For one thing, as I just explained, a negative motivator can spark your desire to initiate change. But mostly, in the publishing world, a book called* Enjoy Healthy Eating *just doesn't have the same impact. So forgive us for that.*

With Charlie, who was fully determined to conquer his emotional overeating problem NOW, I used another set of techniques called Time Empowerment Techniques®, which you'll learn about in chapter 8. After we did this work, I had him redo his list of values, and I can tell you that the list was very different from his first list. They were not only positive statements on the surface level, but the underlying motivators no longer contained an 'away from.' This meant that his motivators and values would continue to be applicable after he reached his goal weight.

With this in mind, go back to the list you created. Notice how many of them contain negative motivators that are driving you away from what you don't want? Write "away from" next to each of these. If you have a lot of negative motivators, it may be an indicator that more advanced work on your values, like the type of work I did with Charlie in the office, may be useful for you. In addition, in advanced values work, we also pay attention to the sequence of your values, and are able to change them to align with your eventual goals of what you want.

Now, take some time to think again about what is important to you about being healthy. Think in positive terms that are helping you get what you want, not negative terms that are getting you away from what you don't want.

For example, is it important to you to:

- *Feel happy?*
- *Enjoy emotional stability?*
- *Feel calm and confident?*
- *Have great energy?*
- *Be a great role model for my children?*
- *Love myself?*
- *Participate in sports and other activities I love?*
- *Enjoy taking on new challenges?*

Write down what is driving your desire to change. If you notice that it is very difficult to use positive language here, it may indicate that doing some change work on your values, like what Charlie did, would be extremely important and beneficial for you to end your emotional overeating.

Why I Want to Get Healthy, Revisited

_____

_____

_____

_____

_____

_____

_____

For me, my family is my motivation. I have an amazing wife, four wonderful children, and a new grandson, Elias. My grandfather was one of the most important people in my life. I was named after him and he was my best friend growing up. I know how important grandparents can be. The day Elias was born I thought about my grandfather all day long.

I *want* to be healthy to be able to love Elias like my grandfather loved me. When I really think about what's important to me, it motivates me to eat brain healthy foods, exercise, manage my stress, and do all the things that will help me live a long life so I can be there for my family and loved ones.

If your motivation involves the ones in your life, put up their pictures where you can see them every day. This is my screensaver.

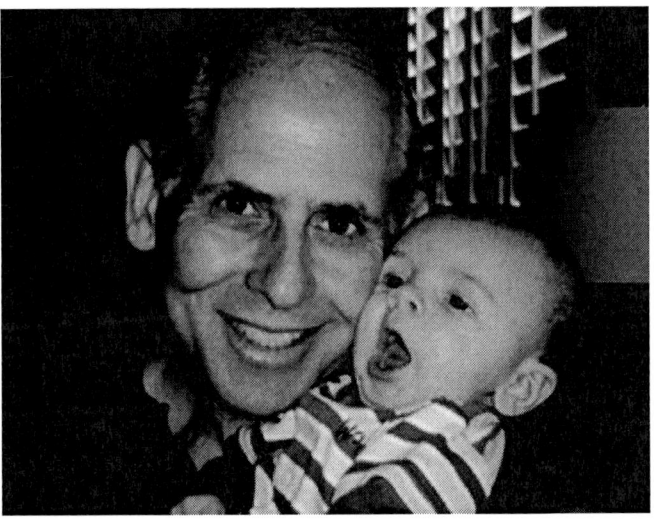

As I was writing End Emotional Overeating NOW with Daniel, I had the opportunity to think about my own values and motivators to get healthy. I eat an overall very healthy diet, mostly vegan, with hardly any unnecessary or added sugars, fats, or salt. However, extra caffeinated chai tea was one of my vices. You have to understand, I have been drinking one cup of tea with breakfast every single day of my life since

high school. It makes me feel good and ready to start my day.

However, when I started medical school, the long hours really got to me and I started drinking additional cups of tea throughout the day. I especially believed that the extra tea could give me the additional energy I needed to make it through the 24- to 36-hour shifts I greatly disliked during residency training when I was "on call." After all, who doesn't need a little pep when you are being woken up at 3 a.m. to handle a call from the emergency room?

That habit of drinking chai tea throughout the day stuck with me long after I graduated from my residency training. Here at Amen Clinics, I would have a cup with breakfast, another cup mid-morning, and sometimes another cup after lunch. Recently, I noticed that at the end of the day when I wanted to focus on writing, I was experiencing fuzzy thinking, a lack of focus, a mild headache and a lot of tension. I thought I needed to drink even more *tea to make my thinking clearer and for my headache to go away.*

Ironically, as a psychiatrist at Amen Clinics, where we specialize in brain imaging, I mentally knew that too much caffeine vaso-constricts and thereby reduces blood flow to the brain. But I didn't think that was what was happening to me! After all, I'm only drinking three cups a day, I thought to myself. Nevertheless, I decided to find out if that might be the problem.

I made a conscious decision to end my relationship with the extra cups of tea. Because I didn't want to give up my morning tea with breakfast, just the other cups during the day, I didn't use Like to Dislike, which I talk about in chapter 7. The first few days, I felt very fatigued, as if I wanted to take a nap in the afternoon. I thought about how much I wanted some tea—to taste it and to feel the warm cup in my hands.

But after several days, I could tell that the tension I had been feeling was dissipating, my thinking was sharper, and I felt more focused. The extra tea really was what was making me feel so lousy. And I finally realized just how lousy I was feeling.

This is something I often emphasize with my patients—that they may not understand the far-reaching negative effects of their emotional overeating or other detrimental behaviors until they actually stop *the behavior.*

Getting through the first week wasn't easy, but I wrote a list of what was motivating me to stop drinking the tea and referred to it whenever I felt like I wanted to drink some tea. Here are my positive motivators on the list:

- *I care about my brain health.*
- *I want to be focused.*
- *I want to think clearly.*
- *I want to be tension-free.*
- *I want to be a good role model for my patients.*
- *I want to live with integrity and live the positive messages I tell my patients every day.*

This list helped me stick with it and stop drinking the tea. With time, I am creating a new healthy habit by building a new neurological circuitry that is going to be good for me. This idea of a new circuitry is something I also like to educate my patients about, especially after we do any kind of change work.

Do You Believe?

If you want to end emotional overeating NOW, you *must* believe you can do it. At the very least, you have to believe that there is a *possibility* that you can change. Without this belief, it is unlikely you will succeed in ending emotional overeating on a long-term basis. Believing that this program can work for you is also essential.

How do you find that belief? Our hope is that this program and the many success stories it contains will infuse you with the belief that you can do it, too. We have seen this program work for so many people, and we know it can work for you too… if you believe in yourself. Take Rick, for example, who attended the taping of my latest public television special,

The Amen Solution. Rick sent me an email with the subject line "Someone flipped a switch in my brain." Here's what he wrote:

> Dr. Amen:
>
> I wanted to let you know of an exciting change in my life since the taping of your new public television special. In the five or six weeks since the live recording, I've lost 30 pounds, and counting.
>
> At the time of the taping I had over 350 pounds weighing down my frame. Fast food was a staple of my diet, and portions were always big. Despite the large amount of food I'd take in daily, I had regular cravings for more of the same. I loved the "high" that came with double-cheeseburgers for dinner and ice cream for dessert.
>
> After your program I honestly didn't expect a life change. I knew myself too well—impulsive, no willpower, and no endurance. A couple years ago I had given some serious effort to losing weight and changing my eating habits, but it was like going through boot camp, and I couldn't keep it up.
>
> But in the days following your program's taping, a co-worker of mine decided to follow the 10th Solution you offered: "Influence others to be thinner, smarter, and happier..." He told me he'd join me in enacting a healthy lifestyle, in line with the principles you laid out.
>
> My coworker then showed me before-and-after photos of a friend of his who had lost more weight than I was hoping to lose (150 pounds). The key to his sustained weight loss was a lifestyle change, not a fad diet.
>
> That was all I needed. Suddenly it was no longer impossible, it was *inevitable*. I knew I was going to

lose this weight.

With the help of my coworker and the partnership of my wife in this new path, I traded the fast food in for more nutritious options. At first I was very fearful that I wouldn't be satisfied, or that my cravings would just drive me back to the same old foods and huge portions. But something amazing happened—my cravings disappeared virtually *overnight*. I had no idea that nutritious foods could be so satisfying! It's like someone flipped a switch in my brain!

Since that very first day I haven't felt cheeseburgers calling my name. My portions are way down (another thing I did not expect), and I have had full and consistent energy every day. In truth, this has been far easier than I anticipated. It now feels completely natural to me to eat this way, to think about what I'm putting in my body, and to feel good about making wiser food choices. I don't feel the least bit deprived (I'll have the occasional burger, but now it's a low-fat salmon or buffalo burger). At last I've found something I can do for the rest of my life, and the benefits, though obvious, have only just begun.

About a year from now I'll be at my ideal size. But I'm in no rush. I'm having a great time getting there!

Thanks for inspiring my coworker. In my case, it made all the difference.

Rick

Rick's story is so amazing. Realizing that somebody else believed in him helped Rick believe in himself. Here's why Larry thinks this is so important.

Rick's inspiring story is also an example of an important concept I call using positive emotions to support you in ending emotional overeating versus letting negative emotions get in the way. Here's what I mean by that. When Daniel does his public television special, it is reaching people in a positive way. This is, in a sense, instilling positive emotion into people to help them on their path towards ending emotional overeating.

When you combine that with positive emotional support from friends and family, it becomes a very powerful motivator. In fact, it is very much like the power of suggestion or even hypnosis. You hear the other people telling you that you can do it, and you start to believe it and act on it.

Here's another example of how positive reinforcement from others helps you believe in your ability to change.

My best friend, let's call him Jason, used to love French fries. He always ordered fries with his meals and couldn't get enough of them. Even if he had already eaten dinner and saw a plate of fries, he would eat them even though he was full.

Jason and I were having dinner together one night and he told me he wanted to look good in his tuxedo for his upcoming wedding. I asked him if he wanted help to stop eating French fries, and he said okay.

Using just a napkin and a pen, it took only 15 minutes to get him to stop wanting to eat fries. The next day, he texted me to say that someone in his office had brought him some French fries and he felt repulsed by them and pushed them away. "This is unbelievable!" he texted.

Four months later, he still hasn't eaten a single fry. His family, who used to cater to Jason's love of fries, started bringing him salads instead. Every time they bring him a salad now, it is positive support that serves as positive reinforcement to stay on the path to reach his goal.

Who are the people that believe in you? What are the things that fill you with belief? Create a list of people, books, songs, and anything else that makes you believe in your ability to change your ways.

My Believe List

_____

_____

_____

_____

Are You Ready to Let Go and Willing to Do What it Takes?

We have both met with patients who have told us that they are very motivated to get their emotional overeating under control and then say, "Okay, doc, go ahead and fix me." Unfortunately, that's not the way it works. We can help facilitate change, but we cannot change you or "fix" you. You are the key to your success, and you have to be an active part of the process.

To end emotional overeating NOW, you have to be both ready and willing to change. Being ready to change but unwilling to do what it takes isn't enough. Likewise being willing to do the work but not quite ready to break up completely with the foods that have you in their grips won't cut it. Approaching this with anything less than a 100 percent commitment is setting yourself up for less-than-optimal results. In fact, if I notice that someone isn't 100% committed to making a change, I gently suggest to them to come back at another time in the future when they are ready and willing to.

Are You Ready and Willing Quiz
Answer yes or no to the following.

1. Are you hoping you can still eat your emotional trigger foods, just in smaller amounts? _____

2. Are you anticipating having "cheat days" but only when you're

really, really stressed out or upset? ____

3. Is it impossible for you to envision yourself in a stressful or sad situation and not turning to food for comfort? ____

4. Are you hoping you can end emotional overeating without making much of an effort? ____

If you answered "no" to all four questions, you are likely ready and willing to end emotional overeating. If you answered "yes" to any of the above questions, you may still be on the fence about changing your behavior. Keep reading to discover the tools that can help you change and to start envisioning a new way of thinking about food and dealing with your emotions. Then retake this test after completing this program.

Staying Motivated

Finding what motivates you to end emotional overeating is one thing. Staying motivated throughout your journey is another. One of the keys to staying motivated is finding something you can be passionate about that keeps you feeling energized and excited… something other than food. What are things that interest you in life? Cars? Sports? Music? Reading? Animals? Dancing? Your kids? Spirituality? Engage in these activities as often as you can. When you feel sad, mad, nervous, or afraid, turn to these activities rather than food to help you deal with your emotions. In the space below, write down all the things you love.

Non-Food Things I Love

_____

_____

_____

_____

One-Page Miracle

One of the most powerful yet simple exercises we use at Amen Clinics is called the One-Page Miracle. It will help guide nearly all of your thoughts, words, and actions. It is called the One-Page "Miracle" because it can quickly focus and change people's lives. It is particularly effective for people who want to lose weight because it makes you focus on what is truly important to you and forces you to think about long-term goals rather than just the immediate gratification that comes from mindless eating or bingeing.

As you will see, this exercise asks you to include your hopes and dreams for four specific areas—biological, psychological, social, spiritual. That is because emotional overeating isn't simply an eating problem. There can be biological factors, psychological reasons, social issues, and spiritual troubles contributing to your problem. In order to break free from the emotional issues that are leading you to overeating, you need to address all four areas.

Directions: Use the following "My One-Page Miracle" or the One-Page Miracle maker on our website, write out what's important to you in each of the areas listed. Be sure to write what you want, not what you don't want. Be positive and use the first person. Write what you want with confidence and the expectation that you will make it happen. Use SMART goals (Specific, Measurable, Attainable, Realistic, and Timely).

When you've finished, place this piece of paper where you can see it every day, such as on your refrigerator, by your bedside, or on the bathroom mirror. In that way, every day you focus your eyes on what's important to you. This makes it easier to match your behavior to what you want. Your life becomes more conscious and you spend your energy on goals that are important to you.

Here is an example from an emotional overeater who was suffering from depression. Zoe, 31, started binge eating in high school when her boyfriend dumped her. That started a pattern of bingeing whenever she felt sad or stressed, like when she didn't get chosen by the sorority she had pledged and when she got passed over for a promotion at work. Even though she had gained more than 60 pounds since high school and couldn't look at herself in the mirror, she couldn't stop her secret bingeing. She avoided dating because she didn't see how any man could find her attractive, and she was so depressed about her weight that she had stopped participating in activities she used to enjoy, like playing piano.

Zoe's brain SPECT scans showed too much activity in the deep limbic system, which is involved with mood, motivation, and appetite. They also revealed an overactive anterior cingulate gyrus, which is common in people who get stuck on thoughts, such as thoughts about food. It is also common in people with binge eating disorders.

After you look at the example, fill out the OPM for yourself.

Sample One-Page Miracle
ZOE'S ONE-PAGE MIRACLE

BIOLOGICAL—to be the healthiest I can be
Brain health: To love my brain starting TODAY, and before I do anything I will think about how it will affect the health of my brain.
Physical health: To make an appointment with my doctor next week to check my important health numbers and to optimize anything that is out of whack.
Eating: To eat only nutritious foods that provide healthy fuel for my brain, body, and emotions and to be mindful of what I am eating and why.
Weight: To lose 1-2 pounds per week for the next ten weeks.
Exercise: To do 30 minutes of fast walking four times a week.

PSYCHOLOGICAL—to love myself, respect myself, and be forgiving of myself
Emotional health: To exercise and take fish oil and SAMe to deal with my depression and to practice healthier ways to deal with stress.
Thinking patterns: To question my ANTs (automatic negative thoughts), focus on the positive, believe in myself, and be grateful every day.

SOCIAL—to be connected to those I love and to develop a strong support group
Relationships: To open myself up to dating and new relationships.
Children: No children now, but when I do have kids, I want to be a great role model.
Support: To join an online weight-loss community this week and ask my family to support me in my efforts.
Work/Money: To feel more confident about myself so I can apply for the outside sales job at work.

SPIRITUAL—to feel connected to a higher power and others
Spirituality: To meditate daily.
Passions: To start playing the piano again by taking piano lessons once a week.
Meaning: To make a difference in someone else's life today.

MY ONE-PAGE MIRACLE
What Do I Want? What Am I Doing To Make It Happen?

BIOLOGICAL

Brain health: _____

Physical health: _____

Eating: _____

Weight/exercise: _____

PSYCHOLOGICAL

Emotional health: _____

Thinking patterns: _____

SOCIAL

Significant other: _____

Children: _____

Support: _____

Work/money: _____

SPIRITUAL

Spirituality: _____

Passions: _____

Meaning: _____

Chapter 4

CORRECT NEGATIVE THOUGHTS

*Change Your Thinking to Change Your
Eating Habits*

One of the most powerful techniques you can use to stop emotional overeating is to get control of your mind and stop believing every illogical, irrational, ridiculous thought that goes through your head.

Your thoughts can lie. They may lie a lot, and it is often these deceptive thoughts that drive your anxiety, sadness, and anger that lead to emotional overeating.

Brain imaging shows us that negative thinking has a negative effect on brain function that sours your mood, slows your thinking process, and makes you more impulsive—*I need the pizza now!* A study we conducted at Amen Clinics clearly shows that negative thinking dramatically decreases activity in the cerebellum and temporal lobes.

Decreased activity in the temporal lobes is associated with mood problems, temper control problems, and memory loss. Reduced activity in the cerebellum puts the brakes on your thought process and lowers impulse control and coordination.

Talk about a recipe for weight gain! When you feel sad or fly off the handle, you are far more likely to reach for the chips and soda rather than the raw carrot sticks and green tea.

Bad, mad, sad, hopeless, or helpless thoughts also release chemicals that make you feel lousy. Your hands get cold, you start to sweat, your heart rate speeds up, you breathe faster and more shallowly, and your muscles tense up. These awful, miserable, negative thoughts can make you feel anxious, depressed, angry, or despondent and make you run to the refrigerator.

In our weight-loss groups, the vast majority of the participants have absolutely no idea that their thoughts are controlling them and keeping them chained to their emotional overeating. For example, my patient Sheri recently told me that she feels guilty whenever she doesn't clean her plate. When she was a child, her mother made her feel bad if she didn't eat everything she served.

I remember my mom trying to do the same thing to me. "Think about the poor people in China," she said. One of the few times she hit me was when I replied, "Well, let's pack it up and send it to them." The other time she hit me was when I lit the couch on fire when I was five years old. But that is a story for another time.

I asked Sheri to write down the thought, "I should eat everything on my plate."

"Is that true?" I asked

"Of course, it isn't true," she said. "Look at me. It's obvious I have eaten way too much. I am done letting her voice inside my head control me."

Negative Thoughts are ANTs

The thought, "I should eat everything on my plate" is an ANT. ANT stands for automatic negative thoughts, the thoughts that come into your mind automatically and ruin your day.

Emotional overeaters tend to be infested with ANTs. Here are some of the more common ANTs I've heard from my patients who are emotional overeaters. You may have had a few of these thoughts yourself. If so, circle them.

"Food is the only thing that makes me feel good."

> *"I have no control over my eating."*
>
> *"If only I could lose weight, I'd be happy."*
>
> *"I doubt I'll ever be successful at losing weight."*
>
> *"I shouldn't have eaten that. I'm doomed to be fat forever."*

Lies! Lies! Lies! These thoughts are all lies that conspire to keep you chained to emotional overeating. One of the biggest lies I hear from emotional overeaters is some variation of the following:

> *"I'm having such a rotten day, I deserve a treat."*

Larry calls this particular lie the Halloween lie. You think that bingeing on your favorite foods is a treat to reward yourself, but it's actually a trick. Overeating is anything but a treat for your weight, emotional well-being, and happiness. This one scary ANT keeps you mired in your emotional turmoil and keeps you from ever reaching your weight goals.

Carlos knows a lot about ANTs. His mind was filled with worries and negative thinking when he first came to Amen Clinics for help with his anger and trouble focusing. Carlos weighed 266 pounds, in part because whenever he had negative thoughts, he would eat to feel better. "I was always looking for something to make me happy," he said.

By using many of the tools in this program, especially correcting negative thoughts, Carlos lost 50 pounds and noticed a dramatic improvement in his moods, as well as his energy and memory. By learning to kill the ANTs, he no longer overate to medicate his sadness. And by eating brain healthy foods, he no longer had the energy crashes that made him so vulnerable to stress.

On the outside, it is like he is a different person. We saw the same dramatic difference on the inside as well. How cool is that? His brain is dramatically better. By changing his thinking patterns and eating habits, he changed his brain and in the process changed his life!

When we introduce the concept of ANTs to our weight-loss groups, the reaction is amazing. Many of them say it is the single most helpful thing they learn from our program.

Learning to kill the ANTs by challenging your thoughts is critical to winning the battle of the bulge. In this chapter, you will learn how to develop an internal ANTeater to talk back to your negative thoughts so they won't send you racing to the cookie jar. Because getting control of your thinking is so important to your success, be sure to spend ample time completing the exercises in this chapter and make copies of them so you can use them whenever you experience an ANT infestation.

Negative Thoughts are Contagious

I often say that ANTs are contagious. Negative thoughts are like a virus that passes from one person to the next. Turn on the TV, open a newspaper, or check the headlines online, and you'll be bombarded with negative messages that breed fear, anxiety, disgust, and horror. Go to pick up your kids at school and you'll hear parents complaining about the teachers, the parking, and the other parents. At work, you'll get an earful of negativity from your co-workers who bad-mouth each other any chance they get.

Even your friends and family may be part of the problem. While I was recently on tour for one of my public television shows, I met with one of my favorite co-hosts who was overweight. As we were talking at a break, she told me that she often went out to eat with her friends, always to places with "the unhealthiest food." She said it was her only social time and even though she wanted to lose weight, she was afraid of losing the social connections.

I asked her if she really thought it was true, that if she didn't eat at unhealthy places, she would have no friends. Sheepishly she smiled. She had been watching my programs for years. "That is an ANT," she said. "If I believe that thought, then I am doomed to only eat at bad places. I am giving myself permission to die early."

With a simple question and a nudge, she got the concept. She did not have to believe every irrational thought that was keeping her trapped in unhealthy restaurants. If these ladies were really her friends, they could choose healthier places to socialize, or she needed a new group of friends. Are your friends' bad habits or negative thoughts killing you?

Meet the ANTs

Over the years, therapists have identified ten "species" of ANTs or types of negative thoughts that keep you chained to emotional overeating:

1. All or nothing
2. Always thinking
3. Focusing on the negative
4. Thinking with your feelings
5. Guilt beating
6. Labeling
7. Fortune telling
8. Mind reading
9. Blame
10. Denial

1. All or nothing

Here, people think that things are all good or all bad. One of the people I met on a recent public television show tour told me she hated the gym so much that she would never exercise. I asked her, "Do you like to dance?" She replied, "Oh, I love to dance." "How about taking a walk on the beach?" I asked. "I like that, too," she said. When I told her that dancing and walking on the beach are forms of exercise, she gave me a puzzled look. She had always equated "exercise" only with the gym.

When she realized that any type of physical activity qualified as a type of exercise, she said, "Maybe I don't hate to exercise; maybe I just hate the gym." This is an example of all or nothing thinking, when you believe that everything is all good or all bad. It is the same as black-or-white thinking.

Here are a few more examples:

> *"I haven't eaten any chocolate all week, I have got this licked."*
>
> *"I got stressed and ate a doughnut. I am doomed to be fat."*
>
> *"We had an argument that sent me straight to the fridge for a slice of leftover birthday cake. Since I ate one piece, I may as well eat the whole cake."*

Ending emotional overeating takes time, and you will likely run into a few speed bumps and small failures along the way. But that doesn't mean that *you* are a failure. When you find yourself slipping back into your old patterns, take stock of what is going on in your life that you are having trouble dealing with and practice the techniques in this program to help you cope in a more healthy way.

2. Always thinking

This is when you overgeneralize a situation. Always thinking usually involves thoughts with words, such as always, never, every time, or everyone. Here are some examples:

> *"I will never be able to stop eating fried chicken."*
>
> *"I have always been fat; it will never change."*
>
> *"Every time I try to exercise, I get injured."*
>
> *"She's always in a bad mood."*
>
> *"No one ever listens to me."*
>
> *"Every time I get stressed, I have to eat something."*

> *"I don't like any of the foods that are good for me."*

Always thinking ANTs are very common. Beware when they creep into your mind because they can have a very immediate, negative effect on your mood. Plus, they sentence you to a lifetime of overeating and other bad habits.

Always thinking ANTs make you believe you have no control over your actions and behaviors and that you are incapable of changing them. When you find yourself barraged by an always thinking ANT, ask yourself if it is really true. For example, is it true that no one *ever* listens to you? Ever? Think of occasions when people have listened to you to help squash this pesky ANT.

3. Focusing on the negative

So many people who are overweight and unhappy can find something negative to say about any situation no matter how positive it may seem to other people. This ANT can take a positive experience, relationship, or achievement and taint it with negativity. It is the judge, jury, and executioner of new experiences, new relationships, and new habits.

> *"I wanted to lose 30 pounds in ten weeks, but I have only lost 8 pounds. I'm a complete failure."*

> *"When I got stressed last night, I avoided eating chips by going for a walk, but it started to drizzle and ruined my hair so I'm never doing that again."*

> *"I started eating two servings of vegetables a day, but I should be eating five for optimal health, so I should just give up on eating them altogether."*

Focusing on the negative releases brain chemicals that make you feel bad, make you more inclined to give up on your efforts, and set you up for failure.

Try focusing on the positive, and it will improve your mood and make you feel better about yourself. Putting a positive spin on your thoughts leads to positive changes in your brain that make you happier and smarter and will help you end emotional overeating.

For example, here's how you could think about these same situations:

> *"I have already lost 8 pounds and have changed my lifestyle so I will continue to lose weight until I reach my goal of losing 30 pounds."*
>
> *"After walking, I felt energized and proud of myself that I didn't give in to the chips."*
>
> *"Eating two servings of vegetables a day is better than none."*

If you want your brain to work better, be grateful for the good things in your life. At Amen Clinics, we performed a SPECT study, which found that practicing gratitude causes real changes in your brain that enhance brain function and make you feel better. Learning how to spin your negative thoughts into positive ones takes practice. Here are two exercises I recommend.

Gratitude Exercise #1

Write down five things you are grateful for every day. Use the space provided or just use a notepad to write down the things you are grateful for. The act of writing helps to solidify them in your brain. In research from the University of Pennsylvania, doing a similar exercise boosted patients' level of happiness in just three weeks. Doing this exercise every day can be very helpful in ending emotional overeating.

5 Things I'm Grateful For Today

1. _____

2. _____

3. _____

4. _____

5. _____

Gratitude Exercise #2: The Glad Game

No matter what situation you are in, try to find something to be glad about. Think of a time when you were in a difficult or disappointing situation and started to think negatively but then found (or now can see) a "silver lining." Now, try to explain the same situation from a "glad" standpoint. What did you find to be glad about the situation?

Something I'm Glad About

_____

_____

_____

_____

4. Thinking with your feelings

These ANTs occur when you have a feeling about something, and you assume it is correct so you never question it. Feelings are very complex and are often rooted in powerful memories from the past. Feelings can lie, too. These thoughts usually begin with the words "I feel." For example:

"*I feel stupid.*"

"*I feel like a loser.*"

> *"I feel like nobody will ever love me."*
>
> *"I feel hungry and must eat or I will get sick."*
>
> *"I feel like I have to have some chocolate right now!"*

Whenever you have a strong negative feeling, check it out before running to the kitchen, vending machine, or nearest fast-food restaurant for a snack. Look for the evidence behind the feeling. Do you have real reasons to feel that way? Or, are your feelings based on events or things from the past?

5. Guilt beating

Guilt is generally not a helpful emotion. It often backfires and can be counterproductive to your goals. Thinking in words like "should," "must," "ought to," and "have to" are typical with this ANT.

Here are some examples:

> *"I should stop eating sugar."*
>
> *"I have to count my calories."*
>
> *"I ought to go to the gym more."*

What happens when you say these kinds of things to yourself? Do they make you more inclined to cut the sugar, count calories, or hit the gym? I doubt it. It is human nature to push back when we feel like we "must" do something, even if it is something that will benefit us in the end. It is better to replace "guilt beatings" with phrases like "I want to do this," "It fits with my goals to do that," or "It would be helpful to do this."

In the examples above, it would be beneficial to change the phrases to:

> *"It is my goal to stop eating sugar because it will reduce my cravings, prevent energy crashes, diabetes, and inflammation in*

my body and get me off this energy and emotional rollercoaster."

"I want to count my calories because it will help me learn to take control of my eating."

"It is in my best interest to go to the gym because exercising will burn calories and will make me feel better and more energized."

Here's a story from Larry about his patient Sarah who needed help controlling her guilt beating thoughts.

For years, Sarah had been saddled with guilt over a friend who had committed suicide. Sarah hadn't checked on him in his apartment for a few days and had convinced herself that she should have checked on him sooner, even though there was no indication that he needed to be checked on. Her ANT was that, had she checked on him, he would still be alive.

As we were working on this thought, Sarah asked, "But isn't guilt necessary?"

"Of course, there are times when guilt is necessary," I told her. "Guilt helps prevent us from doing something wrong. Here, we're not removing guilt from your psychological repertoire. We're getting rid of unnecessary *guilt and* inappropriate *guilt that doesn't serve you. And the guilt you have over this incident is irrational and fueling your desire to overeat emotionally."*

After working on this thought, Sarah realized that it was a lie, and she was finally able to let go of her guilt. She sighed in relief and said, "It feels so good to be free from this."

6. Labeling

Whenever you call yourself or someone else names or use negative terms to describe them, you have a labeling ANT in your brain. A lot of us do this on a regular basis.

You may have said one of the following at some point in your life:

> *"He's a jerk."*
>
> *"I'm lazy."*
>
> *"I'm a loser."*
>
> *"She's a slob."*
>
> *"I'm a wimp."*

The problem with negative labels is they exercise negative pathways in the brain and make them stronger. Negative pathways can lead to negative behaviors, including the very behaviors you are trying to change. Calling yourself names takes away your control over your thoughts and actions. For example, if you are a "nervous Nelly" then of course you are going to feel anxious. If you are "Mad Mike" then you will live up to that label and blow your top when things don't go your way. If you are a "downer" then you'll never lift your blue moods. It is as if you have given up before you have even tried. This defeatist attitude keeps you stuck in your old ways.

Beware Of The Red ANTs

These last four ANTs are the worst of the bunch. I call them the red ANTs because they can really sting and can prevent you from ending emotional overeating.

7. Fortune telling

Do you tend to predict the worst? If so, you may have a fortune telling ANT infestation. These ANTs can creep into anybody's mind, but they are especially common in emotional overeaters.

> *"I could lose 100 pounds, but I doubt I could maintain it."*

> *"I might be able to diet for a few months, but I can't change my habits forever."*
>
> *"If I get nervous and don't eat, I'll have a panic attack."*

Predicting the worst in a situation causes an immediate rise in heart rate and breathing rate and can make you feel anxious. When you feel like this, it can trigger your cravings for sugar or refined carbs and make you feel like you need to eat to calm your anxiety.

What makes fortune telling ANTs even worse is that your mind is so powerful that it can make happen what you see. For example, when you are convinced that you will have a panic attack, you run that thought through your head over and over and may begin to feel the physical symptoms of a panic attack, making you crave your comfort foods even more.

Similarly, if you are convinced that you won't be able to maintain your weight loss, you will be less likely to adopt brain healthy habits that could help you shed those extra pounds and keep them off. When you have fortune telling ANTS, it keeps you stuck in your old destructive patterns.

8. Mind reading

When you think you know what others are thinking even though they have not told you, and you have not asked them, it is called mind reading. Mind reading is very common, and it can make you feel so awful that you seek out food to soothe the emotional upheaval. Here are some examples of mind reading ANTs:

> *"My boss is mad at me because he didn't say hi to me when he walked by."*
>
> *"She didn't call me today. She probably wants to break up with me."*

"They hate me."

Of course these thoughts are going to make you feel terrible emotionally. And they quickly put you on a downward spiral of negative thinking. When you think the boss is mad at you, you start fretting about what you did wrong at work and start wondering if you'll lose your job, spend all your savings, rack up credit card debt, lose your house, and end up living in your car. It's no wonder you want a cookie to help you feel better.

I have twenty-five years of education—mostly in how to diagnose, treat, and help people—and I can't read anyone's mind. I have no idea what they are thinking unless they tell me. A glance in your direction doesn't mean somebody is talking about you or mad at you. I tell people that a negative look from someone else may be nothing more than his being constipated! You just don't know.

When there are things you don't understand, ask for clarification, and stay away from mind reading ANTs. They are very infectious and can put you in an emotional tailspin.

The Most Dangerous Red ANTs

Of all the ANTs, the blame and denial ANTs are the ones that hurt the most. Having these ANTs roaming around in your mind can prevent you from ever conquering your emotional overeating.

9. Blame

Blaming others for your problems is toxic thinking. When you make excuses and blame others for the problems in your life, you become a victim of circumstances, and you cannot do anything to change your situation. It signifies that you think you have no control over your own life, and you aren't taking responsibility for your behavior. People who are infested with blame ANTs tend to make a lot of excuses for their overeating.

Be honest with yourself and ask yourself if you have a tendency to say things like the following:

> "Everybody else at the table was having seconds, and I didn't want to be rude, so I did, too."
>
> "It's not my fault I eat too much; my mom taught me to clean my plate."
>
> "If restaurants didn't serve so much food, I wouldn't be so fat."
>
> "I wouldn't have drunk so much soda, but they kept giving me free refills."
>
> "I will always be fat; it is my genetics."

Whenever you begin a sentence with "It is your fault that I…" it can ruin your life. These ANTs make you a victim. And when you are a victim, you are powerless to change your behavior. To break free from emotional overeating, you have to change your thinking, so kill the blame ANTs, stop making excuses, and start making it your responsibility to change. Take half your entrée to go, say "no" to seconds and free refills, and split restaurant meals with a friend.

And remember, your genes are *not* your destiny. My genes say that I am supposed to be fat, but by eating right, exercising, and practicing brain healthy habits, I'm able to maintain a healthy weight. Research shows that exercise and eating a healthy diet can turn off the "obesity gene."

It is your life. I love what Vernon Howard once wrote, "Permitting your life to be taken over by another person is like letting the waiter eat your dinner." It just makes no sense.

10. Denial

In an Australian study, individuals with a BMI between 30 and 40, which is in the obese range, believed they could lose weight if they needed to, but they didn't feel it was necessary! Talk about denial.

Emotional overeaters are often filled with denial ANTs like these:

> *"I never really feel sad, so I can't be an emotional overeater."*
>
> *"Everybody eats in secret. There's nothing wrong with it."*
>
> *"I only binge when I'm very stressed out, so it isn't a problem."*

The first example above is something I hear from several of my overweight patients. With these patients, whenever feelings of sadness arise in them, they stuff those emotions back down with food so quickly that they don't even realize that they were feeling sad. They don't connect the sadness with the intense cravings they experience. This can also occur with any other emotion, such as anger, fear, or anxiety.

Until you admit that you have a problem, you will be unsuccessful in overcoming emotional overeating.

Kill the ANTs to Take Control of Your Thoughts and Emotions

Now that you are familiar with the various species of ANTs, it is time to learn how to kill the pesky thoughts. With the ANT-killing exercises in this chapter, you will discover how to turn your negative thinking into positive, accurate, healthy thinking. Did you know that happy, positive, hopeful, loving thoughts release chemicals that make you feel good? Scientific studies have found that changing your thinking can be as effective as antidepressant medications to treat anxiety and depression.

Take note, I am not recommending pie-in-the-sky happy, delusional thinking. What I want you to adopt is *honest* thinking. Honest thinking can help you feel happier, think more clearly, and keep you healthier.

Strong scientific evidence shows that the ANT therapy you will learn in this chapter helps with weight loss. Researchers from Sweden found that the people who were trained to talk back to their negative thoughts lost 17 pounds in ten weeks and continued to lose weight over eighteen months, proving this technique works long term. And a 2010 study found that a twelve-week program designed to change thinking patterns helped binge eaters stop bingeing for at least one year.

Develop an internal ANTeater that kills the negative thoughts that come into your head and mess up your life. Teach your ANTeater to talk back to the ANTs so you can free yourself from negative thinking patterns.

Whenever you feel sad, mad, nervous, obsessive, or out of control, write down the thoughts that are going through your mind. The act of writing them down helps to get them out of your head. Identify the ANT species, then talk back to them. Challenging negative thoughts takes away their power and gives you control over your thoughts, moods, and behaviors.

ANT-Killing Examples

ANT	Species of ANT	Kill the ANT
I'm always starving.	Always thinking	Am I really *starving*? No, maybe I'm just eating because I'm bored.
If I lose weight, I'll never be able to keep it off.	Fortune telling	I don't know that. If I change my habits I may be able to maintain my weight loss.
I'm a wreck.	Labeling	I'm not perfect, but there are many things I do well.
It's your fault I eat too much.	Blame	I need to take responsibility for what I eat.

My ANTeater Chart

Whenever you feel sad, mad, nervous, obsessive, bored, or out of control, use the following chart to write out your thoughts and talk back to them. You can also find interactive ANT-killing exercises on our website.

ANT	Species	ANTeater
_____	_____	_____
_____	_____	_____
_____	_____	_____
_____	_____	_____

Do "The Work®"

One of my favorite books, *Loving What Is*, comes from a close friend Byron Katie. In this very wise book, Katie, as her friends call her, describes an amazing transformation that took place in her own life. At the age of forty-three, Katie, who had spent the previous ten years of her life in a downward spiral of rage, addiction, despair, and suicidal depression, woke up one morning on the floor of a halfway house to discover that all those horrible emotions were gone. In their place were feelings of utter joy and happiness.

Katie's great revelation, which came in 1986, was that it is not life that makes us feel depressed, angry, abandoned, and despairing, rather it is our thoughts that make us feel that way. This insight led Katie to the notion that our thoughts could just as easily make us feel happy, calm, connected, and joyful.

It also led her to realize that our minds and our thoughts affect our bodies. "The body is never our problem. Our problem is always a thought that we innocently believe," she wrote in her book *On Health, Sickness, and Death*. In the same book, she also wrote, "Bodies don't crave, bodies don't want, bodies don't know, don't care, don't get hungry or thirsty. It is what that mind attaches—ice cream, alcohol, drugs, sex, money—that the body reflects. There are no physical addictions, only mental ones. Body follows mind. It doesn't have a choice."

Katie also writes, "It's only when I believe a stressful thought that I get hurt. And I'm the one who's hurting me by believing what I think. This is very good news, because it means that I don't have to get someone else to stop hurting me. *I'm the one* who can stop hurting me. It's within my power."

Katie wanted to share her revelation with others to help them end their suffering by changing their thinking. She developed a simple method of inquiry called The Work® to question our thoughts. The Work® is simple and very effective, which is why I love it. It consists of writing down any bothersome, worrisome, or negative thoughts, then asking ourselves four questions, and then doing a turnaround. The four questions are:

1. Is it true? (Is the negative thought true?)

2. Can I absolutely know that it is true?

3. How do I react, what happens when I believe that thought?

4. Who would I be without the thought? Or how would I feel if I didn't have the thought?

After you answer the four questions, you take your original thought and turn it around to its opposite, and ask yourself whether the opposite of the original thought is true. Then, turn the original thought around and apply it to yourself (how does the opposite of the thought apply to me personally?). Then, turn the thought around to the other person if the thought involves another person (how does the opposite apply to the other person?). Take time and meditate on each of your answers.

I have done The Work® myself many, many times, and it helped me get through a very painful period of grief. When I did The Work®, I immediately felt better. I was more relaxed, less anxious, and more honest in dealing with my own thoughts and emotions. Now, I always carry the four questions with me, and I use them a lot in my practice and with my friends and family.

I recommended the book to Larry several years ago, and he ended up signing up for a nine-day course with Byron Katie. He found the experience extremely enlightening and has been using The Work® in his practice ever since.

During the nine-day course with Byron Katie, I realized that stressful thoughts are not always true and that questioning them loosens their emotional power over you. I found The Work® so powerful that I have been using it with my patients ever since to help them dismantle their stressful thoughts.

So many of my patients think they are the only ones who are haunted by these thoughts, but I reassure them that there are no new stressful thoughts. It's the same thoughts that tend to recycle repeatedly, including thoughts like "I'm not good enough," "I can't do this," "She doesn't love me," and "No one understands me." We've all had these thoughts at some point. Even me.

I've used The Work® for myself as a process of soul searching, and it really works. Some of the most beautiful moments of my life have occurred when I realized that something I had believed for so many years wasn't true.

It's incredible what happens when part of your stressful "story" falls apart—whether it's that you're not good enough or that you don't deserve success. It's like a little crack in your mind opens up and you begin to experience the opposite of that stressful thought: "I am good enough" or "I do deserve success." All of a sudden, that false premise you had been carrying around for so long falls away, and you feel so much better.

Take your time when you do The Work®. When I do The Work® with a patient, I may spend as much as fifty minutes working on one single stressful thought that carries great power over the person. When you dig deep into the questions and reflect honestly on your responses, the results can be truly life-changing.

The following is an example of how I used the four questions with one of my patients, Michael, to work on one of his negative thoughts. Michael was more than 100 pounds overweight and felt confident that he could lose weight, but doubted that he would be able to keep it off. Use this as an example of how you can use The Work® to kill the ANTs that are keeping you in chains.

Example of The Work®

Negative Thought: "I doubt I can keep the weight off."

Question #1: Is it true that you can't keep the weight off?

"I doubt it," he said.

Question #2: Can you absolutely know that it is true that you can't keep the weight off?

"Yes," Michael replied. He then began to discuss his rationale why he absolutely believed this to be a true fact.

At this point, I directed Michael to stay within the four questions and reminded him that questions 1 and 2 are simple "yes" or "no" questions. When your mind starts using explanations, such as "but" or "because," it is creating rationalizations and justifications, which is stepping outside of The Work® and the four questions. Keep your answers to a simple "yes" or "no."

Question #3: How do you react, what happens, when you believe the thought "I doubt I can keep the weight off?"

Michael said he felt like a failure, like he was doomed to be overweight forever. When I asked him what else happens to him, he said that he can only see himself as being overweight and that makes him give up on his diet and exercise plan. He begins to feel hopeless, and all of that makes him relapse into overeating.

Then I asked Michael how he treats other people when he has that thought. He said he hates other people and is resentful of thin people. He feels mad at his parents for feeding him so much food when he was growing up.

When working on question 3, I also usually ask, "Whose business are you in? (Your business? God's business? The other person's business?) In this case, he was in his own business.

Question 3 of The Work® has an additional dozen or so sub-questions, which are very helpful in going deeper. If your answer to question 3 took less than a minute to answer, or was just 'on the surface' of your thinking, I strongly encourage using the sub-questions, which you can find on Byron Katie's website (www.thework.com).

Question #4: Who would you be without the thought "I doubt I can keep the weight off?"

I encouraged him to stop for a moment and imagine what his life would look like if it weren't even humanly possible to think this thought. I encouraged him to sit very still and really see himself without being able to think that thought. To help Michael envision his life without this thought, I asked him to think back to the first time he had this thought. Michael said it was back in high school when other students made fun of him for being fat. The virus of that thought had stuck with him for thirty years and made him into who he is today.

Then I asked him, "Who were you before that thought occurred to you?"

He said, "I was a happy teenager."

After remembering what his life was like before he had that original thought, he replied that if he didn't have that thought he would be freer and at peace.

I then pointed out to him that the only difference between the way he felt in question 3 and the way he felt in question 4 was a thought. A thought was the only thing making him feel hopeless in question 3, and the absence of that thought was making him feel free and at peace.

Turnaround: What is the opposite thought of "I doubt I can keep the weight off?" Is this thought true or truer than the original thought?

Michael said, "I have no *doubt I can keep the weight off," and he gave several reasons why he had no doubt that he could do it.*

Michael came up with several other possible turnarounds and I encouraged him to think about them and give three examples of how each of them was as true or truer than his original thought.

Here are the turnarounds he came up with:

"*I doubt I* can't *keep the weight off.*"

"*I doubt I can keep the weight* on*.*"

"*I doubt* my thinking *can keep the weight off.*"

These turnarounds require you to be open and creative with your thinking. For example, with this last turnaround, wasn't it really Michael's thinking that was heavy and sluggish? And doesn't he want his thinking to be lean and have energy?

Doing the turnarounds gave him a new perspective on his previously stressful thought and eliminated its powerful effect on him.

The Work® Exercise

Do the following The Work® exercise (based on the teachings of our good friend Byron Katie) every day to investigate and turn around the negative thoughts and beliefs that fuel anxiety, depression, and overeating. Doing The Work® helps you see the truth of your life so clearly that negative emotions and thoughts have no choice but to disappear. What a comfort! Important: You must complete at least seventy written exercises in order to rewire your brain so that you start seeing reality for what it is, instead of telling yourself lies. If you do The Work® once a day, then you need to do it for ten weeks to effectively retrain your brain and change your thinking patterns. You can also do interactive exercises using The Work® on our website.

Write down the negative/stressful thought or belief:

_____

1. Is it true? Close your eyes, be still, and breathe deeply as you contemplate your answer. If your answer is no, continue to Question 3.

Yes _____ No _____

2. Can you absolutely know that it's true? (Can you know more than God/reality?)

Yes _____ No _____

3. How do you react, what happens, when you have the thought? (When you believe that thought?) Pay attention to your body, mind, heart, and self-esteem. Ask yourself whose business you're in when you have the thought—yours, God's, or the other person's. What happens to you physically when you believe the thought? How do you treat others when you believe the thought? How do you treat yourself when you believe the thought? Can you think of any peaceful reason to hold onto the thought? Find more sub-questions at www.thework.com.

_____

_____

_____

4. Who would you be without the thought? How would you feel or live life differently if you didn't believe the thought? Think back to the first time you had the thought and remember what your life was like before you had the thought.

___

___

___

Turn the thought around. Statements can be turned around to yourself, to the other, to the opposite, and to "my thinking" wherever it applies. Find a minimum of three genuine examples in your life where each turnaround is as true or truer than your original statement.

___

___

___

___

___

___

___

Chapter 5

MANAGE YOUR STRESS

*Meditation and Deep-Breathing
Exercises to Calm Stress*

When you get stressed, do you calm your nerves with ice cream, chips, or cheeseburgers? It's no wonder. Some foods, especially those filled with simple carbohydrates like cookies, cake, or bread boost a chemical in our brains called serotonin that can quickly make us feel less anxious and less depressed. The problem is that these comfort foods can become addictive and cause us to lose control. They can lead to imbalances in the brain that make you want to eat more and more and more.

Plus, chronic stress raises levels of the hormone cortisol, which constricts blood flow to the brain and lowers overall brain function. Chronic exposure to stress hormones affects the brain's memory centers as well as an area called the amygdala, which is part of the emotional brain. As a result, chronic stress has negative consequences for your emotional balance.

It's a vicious cycle: you feel stressed all the time, which negatively affects the emotional brain, which puts you on more of an emotional rollercoaster. Then the stress and emotions are so bothersome, you munch on candy to make yourself feel better, but the sugar, fat, and salt work on the heroin centers of your brain and make you addicted to the candy so you eat more of it. Then you watch as your waistline expands and your self-esteem shrinks.

Rest assured there are better ways to deal with stress. Meditation and deep breathing are simple techniques that I use whenever I feel stressed or out of control, and that Larry and I have both been using for years with our patients. There is very good scientific evidence that when you add meditation to a healthy weight-loss program you improve the outcome!

How Meditation Helps Ease Emotional Overeating

Meditation is a wonderful tool to calm your mind and boost your brain at the same time. Meditation actually fooled us. In 2009, we published a scientific study on meditation, and we initially thought it would calm brain activity. But our study showed that a very simple twelve-minute meditation actually boosted blood flow to the prefrontal cortex, the same area of the brain that helps you focus and make good decisions.

I recently treated a woman who was in a severe car accident. Shortly thereafter she had problems with depression, anger, and emotional overeating. Once I taught her to meditate using the same twelve-minute protocol, she noticed that within a month her moods, emotions, and eating behaviors were under much better control.

Decades of research have shown that meditation (and prayer) benefits the brain in many ways that can help you end emotional overeating. Here's how.

Meditation reduces stress, soothes anxiety, and fosters relaxation. Brain imaging studies have shown that meditation calms the anterior cingulate and basal ganglia, which diminishes worries and provides a sense of relaxation. A wealth of research indicates that people who meditate regularly have lower levels of stress, anxiety, and worry. Considering that stress is one of the most common triggers for emotional overeating, reducing your stress levels can be vital to changing your eating patterns.

Meditation improves emotional stability and gives you a bigger brain. A 2009 brain imaging study performed at UCLA found that people who meditate on a regular basis have more gray matter in the hippocampus, orbito-frontal cortex, thalamus, and left inferior temporal gyrus than non-meditators. These areas are all involved in emotional regulation, which may explain why meditators tend to have more positive emotions and better control over their emotions. That can be tremendously beneficial for emotional overeaters.

Meditation reduces depression. Meditation improves your sense of psychological well-being and diminishes symptoms of depression. One study used EEG to show that people who meditated for eight weeks experienced changes in cerebral electrical activity that are typically associated with experiencing positive or joyful feelings.

Learning to Meditate is Easy

You don't need to spend three months in India to learn how to meditate. In my clinical practice, I often recommend meditation as an integral part of a treatment plan. Many of my patients have reported back that they feel calmer and less stressed after just a few minutes of daily meditation.

The following meditation exercises are effective, feel-good techniques to reset your nervous system so that you feel ever so much more relaxed. It is very powerful. You can do this whenever you feel stressed, anxious, or sad.

For example, you can close your office door and take an inner journey on your afternoon break instead of heading to the vending machine. You can do this to mellow out after a hard day or after your children have gone to bed rather than consoling yourself with a bowl of ice cream. I have even practiced guided imagery and self-hypnosis while sitting on trains, buses, and airplanes.

To help you get the most out of meditation, use the following tips and techniques.

Prepare to Meditate

- Find a quiet place that's free of distractions. Lock the door to avoid interruptions and turn off your cell phone.

- Give yourself twelve minutes to meditate, once or twice a day, preferably before breakfast and dinner, and don't stop until this time is up. Check a clock occasionally, or use a soft alarm, not a harsh one, as it might shock you out of your relaxation.

- Sit comfortably and consciously relax all your muscles from the bottom of your feet to the top of your head, and close your eyes. Enjoy your calm attitude as you breathe slowly and deeply from your belly.

- Try to forget all the thoughts that swirl through your mind. Put a stop to your internal monologue. Cease thinking in words. This is often the hardest part about meditation for people who are new to the practice. When memories arise, simply tell them to go away or imagine a broom gently sweeping them out of your mind. With practice, you will find that your thoughts become less intrusive.

Daily Twelve-Minute Kirtan Kriya Meditation Practice

This twelve-minute meditation involves chanting the following simple sounds—"saa" "taa" "naa" "maa"—while doing repetitive finger movements. Do this every day for maximum effect.

- Touch the thumb of each hand to the index finger while chanting "saa."

- Touch the thumb of each hand to the middle finger while chanting "taa."

- Touch the thumb of each hand to the ring finger while chanting "naa."

- Touch the thumb of each hand to the pinkie finger while chanting "maa."

- Repeat the sounds for two minutes aloud.

- Repeat the sounds for two minutes whispering.

- Repeat the sounds for four minutes silently.

- Repeat the sounds for two minutes whispering.

- Repeat the sounds for two minutes aloud.

- When you finish, sit quietly for a minute or two, and try to merge your calmed mind and body with your regular mode of being.

Kirtan Kriya Fingertip Movements

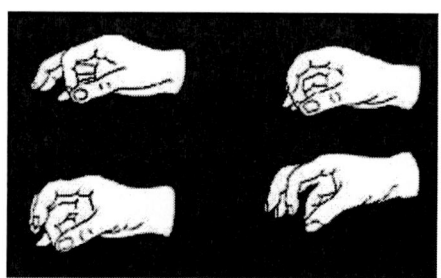

I realize that many people are busy and some days, you just can't find the time to meditate for twelve minutes. Or when you are first trying meditation, you may find it difficult to focus your mind for twelve minutes. In either case, you may want to try meditative deep breathing. In just a few minutes a day, it can help you feel more calm and relaxed.

Meditative Deep Breathing for Stress Relief

Breathing is one of the most vital parts of our lives, yet most of the time, our conscious mind is not even aware that we are breathing. Most people tend to take rapid, shallow breaths, especially when we are stressed. That's because as part of the body's natural stress response, your breathing becomes more shallow.

When you take shallow breaths, it reduces the amount of oxygen that reaches your brain cells, reducing overall brain function. The simple act of breathing also serves to eliminate waste products, such as carbon dioxide, from the body, and shallow breathing can lead to a buildup of carbon dioxide. When there is too much carbon dioxide in your system, it can cause stressful feelings of disorientation and panic, which can lead to emotional overeating.

Diaphragmatic breathing, using the big muscle between your chest and abdominal cavity called the diaphragm, is a relaxation technique that can reverse these effects. Taking deep breaths with your belly also relaxes your muscles, which relieves tension, and helps your brain function more efficiently, which improves your thinking and judgment.

Here's how to breathe from your diaphragm.

Diaphragmatic Breathing Exercise
Practice this simple three-step exercise to learn diaphragmatic breathing.

1. Lie on your back and place a small book on your belly.

2. As you slowly inhale, make the book go up. Hold your breath at the top of the breath for 2 seconds.

3. When you exhale, make the book go down. Hold your breath at the bottom for 2 seconds.

Larry and I both use deep-breathing exercises with our own patients all the time. In fact, Larry teaches a wonderful deep-breathing exercise to his patients, and practiced it in a wellness group he ran at Amen Clinics called *The Path of Wellness*. This life-changing program is designed to reduce stress, enhance relaxation, and promote inner peace. In it, he educated the participants that the process of focusing on your breath is an ancient meditation practice, one that has been done for centuries in the East to bring deep relaxation and peace.

Here is the technique Larry uses.

Stress-Relieving Breathing Strategy

Use this breathing strategy whenever you feel stressed, frustrated, mad, sad, bored, or anxious. You can also use it when you are craving food or whenever you want to feel more relaxed.

- *Start by breathing in through your nose and out through your mouth while pursing your lips. Pursing your lips is important because it helps prevent lightheadedness from hyperventilation, and it also helps with relaxing the muscles in the lungs.*

- *Begin to notice the little gap in between where your inhalation ends and your exhalation begins, and conversely in between where your exhalation ends and your inhalation begins. Just notice it without altering the way you breathe. The gap may only last half a second.*

- *Now, as you are breathing, silently think to yourself, "inhale… gap… exhale… gap… inhale…" in synch with your actual breathing pattern.*

- *As you become aware of the gap, change the words you are saying silently to yourself. As you inhale, silently say or think "I am…" and as you exhale, silently say or think "peace." So the eventual silent thinking pattern would go like this: "I am… gap…peace…gap…I am…gap…peace…gap…"*

- *Continue practicing this silently to yourself for 30 seconds to one minute.*

- *Over time with practice, you may notice that the gap begins to become longer and longer without any effort. As you practice this exercise, you will go deeper into a relaxed state, and you will notice that the gap becomes longer naturally.*

- *Extend your practice continuously so that it goes from 1-2 minutes at a stretch to 5-10 minutes in one sitting.*

- *Also begin to have fun and practice this while listening to someone else speak, or while doing your work, and notice the feeling it brings you.*

- *At any time, you can return to your normal regular breathing state.*

The beauty of this very powerful breathing exercise is that it not only reduces stress, but it also provides the mantra or suggestion, "I am peace." By repeating this calming thought to yourself, you begin to embrace it, believe it, and live it. This is so important for emotional overeaters who tend to eat because they are not *at peace.*

My course participants and patients really respond to this deep-breathing exercise. Take Kathy, for example, who said, "The breathing techniques really work and help a lot. If someone is looking for a great way to find peace, this is a great place to start."

Chapter 6

EAT MORE MINDFULLY

Meditate on Your Meals Rather Than Munching Mindlessly

I grew up as one of seven children. At our family dinner table, if you didn't eat fast, you didn't get seconds. This taught me to eat really fast, a habit I had for decades. I would rush through my meals without fully tasting or enjoying what I was eating.

If you can relate, then you need to s-l-o-w down and start eating more mindfully. Mindful eating, which is really a form of meditation, is all about being aware of what you are eating and being 100 percent present in the moment. When you eat mindfully, you typically eat less and enjoy your food more. For emotional overeaters, this is a powerfully healing combination.

Mindful eating also helps you on a biological level. Did you know that when you eat more slowly, your body produces more of the enzymes that help you digest your food and tell you that you are full?

What is Mindful Eating?

Being mindful means paying attention to what you are doing, thinking, feeling, smelling, touching, and tasting in the present moment. This is especially important for those of you who camp out on the couch all evening and devour entire bags of chips, pretzels, or cookies without even realizing it. With mindless eating, it's usually quantity over quality. You don't necessarily enjoy what you're eating, but you want more of it.

By contrast, when you eat mindfully, you meditate on each bite of food and become aware of the smells, tastes, colors, and textures of your food.

You learn to savor each bite. This helps you become more aware of feeling full and stopping before you overeat.

In a study on the effects of mindfulness on binge eating, a group of 18 women diagnosed with binge-eating disorder decreased their number of weekly binges from four to less than two. Fourteen of the women reduced their bingeing so much that they would no longer have met the criteria for binge-eating disorder.

My friend Andy Newberg, M.D., at Thomas Jefferson University, and his collaborator Mark Waldman, a therapist and an Associate Fellow at the Center for Spirituality and the Mind at the University of Pennsylvania, have teamed up to do a SPECT brain study on mindful eating. At the time of this writing, the study is in its earliest stages, and Andy is hesitant to report any specific findings. But he did say that the initial brain scans show that "the brain is different when eating mindfully." That doesn't surprise me at all.

A Meditative, Mindful Eating Exercise

In Larry's *Path of Wellness* group, he led a fascinating session on fasting and meditative eating.

*My aim with this session was to bring conscious awareness to one of the most important aspects of our existence—how we eat. Conscious eating begins from the very moment we have a sensation in our abdomen signaling us with a thought that we may be hungry and therefore, "we need to eat." [Is it true?] We also explored that **how** we eat is equally as important as **what** we eat if we wish to have any sense of health and weight management.*

I invited people to fast for the 24 hours prior to our last session, but only if they wanted to. Of course, I instructed them to check with their doctor first if they had any medical conditions and to take their medications if they were on any, and I told them to drink a lot of water to stay hydrated. Several people in the group agreed to give it a try, and so did I.

I asked the people who were going to fast to keep notes that day. I wanted them to start noticing what happens in the body and mind when they are not eating habitually. I asked them to write down their thoughts, whether they were thinking, "I need to eat," "I'm starving," or even "I'm going to die if I don't eat."

Then I urged them to use the four questions from The Work® to challenge those thoughts.

"I need to eat." Is that true? "No, I don't need to eat. I'm not dying."

"I'm starving." Is that true? "No, I'm not emaciated." [And by the way, most of us have an ample supply of fat storage to keep us alive for quite some time without food!]

"I'm going to die if I don't eat." Is that true? "No, I'm not going to die right now. In fact, I feel alive."

I wanted them to be aware of all emotions and thoughts that came up while they were fasting. And there were a lot of thoughts and emotions. By writing them down and questioning them, they were able to become aware of the things they tell themselves, to unconsciously justify why they eat.

At first, they felt like their minds were gnawing away at them, urging them to give up the fast and indulge. But once they got past their initial discomfort, their minds began to quiet down. For most of them, the fast got easier as the day went on, and they realized that they felt just fine without food. This opened the door to a new perspective on the role of food in their lives.

That night when we had our session, I surprised them all with a catered meal I provided at the end our session. But this meal was not going to be like any meal they had ever had. First, all the foods were vegan, which means there were no animal products. I've been a vegetarian/virtual vegan my entire life, but most of my participants were not, so the foods were new to them. Secondly, I wanted everyone to eat mindfully.

In our culture, we often eat mindlessly. When we're eating, we're usually talking, watching TV, reading the paper, listening to music, working on the computer, or watching a movie. In restaurants, loud music is blasting in our ears as we dive into our food. These all distract us from the eating process and contribute to mindless eating. It's almost as if this is intentional.

For our mindful eating meditation, I instructed everyone to eat in complete silence. I suggested that they savor every aspect of the eating process—smell the aromas, let your mouth water, feel the texture of the food on your tongue, be aware of chewing and swallowing, and notice all the different tastes and flavors. After not eating for 24 hours, they were primed and focused on eating and grateful to have such an abundance of food.

After we ate in total silence, we talked about the fasting and meditative eating experience. One participant named Carmine said he was surprised that he was able to survive the whole day without eating. Another participant Jerri realized that she had been "eating past the moment I was full, eating and drinking when I'm sad, lonely, etc. I realized I often eat out of habit even if I don't feel hungry."

Some people found that by eating mindfully and sensing every morsel on their taste buds, they experienced intense pleasure from eating for the very first time. It was almost as if they had never tasted their food before. They also ate less *food but felt* more *satisfied.*

Some of them admitted to being skeptical about eating vegan foods and had some negative thoughts about it, including "I won't feel full if there isn't any meat" and "I won't like the way it tastes." But since we had devoted a whole session to The Work® earlier in the course, they had learned to question those thoughts, and as predicted, they were not true.

When they released those thoughts and approached the meal with an open mind, they discovered that they loved the vegan foods. One man named Nick said he was shocked to discover that the soy burgers actually tasted like real burgers—only better!

Everybody, including myself, walked out of the session that night with a sense of gratitude for many different reasons.

Mindful Eating Exercise

Plan a mindful eating experience that you can do either alone or with a friend or spouse. If you choose to do this with someone else, remember there is no talking allowed. If you would like to make the experience even more powerful, you may want to consider fasting for up to 24 hours prior to this dining experience. If you do, be sure to drink plenty of water to stay hydrated, and if you take medication or are diabetic, check with your doctor before fasting.

1. Choose a time and place where you can eat without any distractions—no cell phones, no computers, no music, no reading material, no TV, no kids running around, and no dog or cat underfoot. Be sure to give yourself ample time for this exercise because mindful eating takes much longer than your typical eating style.

2. Prepare your plate, make sure you have everything you need, and then sit down at the table.

3. Once you sit down, do not get up for anything.

4. Before you pick up your utensils, breathe in the smell of the food, look at all the colors and textures, and appreciate how beautiful it looks.

5. Let your mouth water.

6. Pick up your fork and take one very small bite of food. Put your fork down. Let the food linger on the front your tongue, then shift it to the side, and finally to the back of your tongue. Notice if the flavor changes depending on where it is on your tongue. (Your tongue is covered in thousands of taste buds that are designed to recognize four basic tastes: sweet, salty, sour, and

bitter. The sweet/salty taste buds are on the front of the tongue, the sour taste buds are on the side, and the bitter taste buds are at the back of the tongue.)

7. Notice if you like or dislike the way the food tastes. (Sometimes, when you eat mindfully, you discover that you don't actually like the foods you crave.)

8. Chew the bite at least twenty times and notice how it feels as you chew. Listen to the sounds of the food as it pops, slurps, or crunches.

9. Swallow.

10. Notice what it feels like as the food travels down your esophagus to your stomach. Pay attention to what happens to the hunger pangs as you eat.

11. Pay attention to any thoughts that arise as you eat. If they are negative or stressful thoughts, ask yourself if they are true.

12. Continue eating in this manner until you are satisfied.

Chapter 7

LIKE TO DISLIKE

Yes, You Can Stop Craving the Foods You Overeat

In our weight-loss groups at Amen Clinics, a lot of the participants are emotional overeaters or are just hooked on one problematic food. Take Joe, for example. He loved cheeseburgers. I mean *really* loved them. He would think about cheeseburgers while driving to work in the morning. If he drove past a fast-food restaurant, he would pull into the drive-thru, order a burger, and devour it before getting to the office. Lunch usually consisted of two burgers loaded with melted cheese. He often called his wife on his way home from work to see if she wanted him to stop on his way home and pick up a few burgers for dinner.

Joe desperately wanted to stop eating cheeseburgers. He knew they weren't good for his health or his waistline. During our weight-loss program, he had already begun to make a lot of healthy changes to his diet. He started eating fruit and yogurt in the morning for breakfast before going to work so he wouldn't be ravenously hungry and tempted to stop for a cheeseburger. He started eating vegetables and lean chicken for dinner. And he was losing weight. But he still craved cheeseburgers and "cheated" on his brain healthy eating plan on a regular basis.

When this is the case with one of our weight-loss participants, we typically ask Larry to come to one of the weight-loss group sessions to do a demonstration. On this particular night, Larry guided Joe through a powerful technique called "Like to Dislike," which is a technique in neurolinguistic programming (NLP). NLP, along with its plethora of tools and techniques, was created in the 1970s by Richard Bandler and John Grinder. Since then, many other practitioners have fine-tuned and added to the repertoire of techniques. These are powerful tools and techniques, and their use is as much a science as an art.

The basic concept of Like to Dislike is simple: you take a food that you know isn't good for you but can't stop eating and replace the way you encode that food in your brain with something you can't stand.

For Joe, the food he disliked most was fish. By the end of the session that night, when Larry asked Joe if he wanted a cheeseburger, Joe turned his head away and asked for a wastebasket because he thought he might get sick. Joe hasn't eaten a single cheeseburger since that night.

What's even better is Joe has absolutely *no desire* to eat cheeseburgers. Most programs that deal with emotional overeating advise you to *avoid* your problem foods so you don't trigger your cravings. But when you change your unconscious mind, you don't have to control the urges and cravings that used to drive you to overeat... because those cravings and urges *are gone*. You are no longer a hostage to the foods you crave, and you stop fighting with yourself.

For example, Joe can drive by a fast-food restaurant without any yearning to pull into the drive-thru. He can go to lunch with his co-workers and watch them eat cheeseburgers without feeling deprived. He's kicked his cheeseburger habit for good.

How cool is that?

Remember, this is the same technique Larry used to help me break up with Rocky Road ice cream, which I wrote about earlier. But I'm not the only one here at Amen Clinics that Larry has helped with this technique. Once our staff discovered that their cravings could potentially be gone in such a short amount of time, they practically started lining up at Larry's office door.

Since he added Like to Dislike to his repertoire of therapeutic tools for emotional overeating, Larry has helped countless people lose their desire for candy, ice cream, bread, birthday cake, coffee, and many other foods. Larry has seen Like to Dislike work so many times, and has used it himself to help him break up with his own personal problem food: sweet potato French fries. He went to another NLP practitioner who facilitated the session, and he hasn't had the desire to eat sweet potato fries since that day. He hasn't eaten sweet potato fries in more than one year, and he is never tempted by them, even though he goes to the same vegan restaurant two to three times a week where he *used to feel compelled* to eat them. Now he orders a side of fresh steamed kale instead.

In this chapter, Larry offers more insight on this technique, and he will take you through his own Like to Dislike session step-by-step so you can see exactly how he did it.

Changing the Way Problem Foods are Encoded in Your Unconscious Mind

People are so amazed when I use Like to Dislike to help them stop overeating a problem food. Sometimes people have been a slave to a food or beverage (remember sixty-seven-year-old Rita, "the Pepsi lady" who had been drinking Pepsi™ every day for fifty-five years?) for so long that they don't think they will ever be able to stop craving it. Then in many cases, by the time they walk out of my office after a single session, their desire for it is completely gone.

How do I know that it's really gone? I often "magically" have some of their favorite food on hand that I can offer to them before they leave so I can evaluate their reaction to it. For example, I did a session with a patient of mine who wanted to stop eating pizza. At the end of our session, she told me she had no desire to eat pizza.

To test it, I went to the office kitchen and pulled a frozen pizza out of the freezer and offered it to her. She told me she felt sick even seeing the package. But even more telling was what she didn't *say. As a Master Practitioner of NLP, I'm trained to pick up on my patients' non-verbal cues, and hers were crystal clear. She instantly recoiled, turned her head away from the pizza box, and turned her nose up as if she were smelling something awful. She hasn't eaten any pizza since that day, over four months ago.*

Typically, Like to Dislike is a technique I use in the office in a one-on-one setting. But that isn't the only way it works. One of the most fascinating Like to Dislike sessions I have ever done involved the weight-loss group at Amen Clinics. I met with about fifty participants in our conference room and worked with Phillip, one of the group members, on giving up his love of chips. By the end of the group meeting, Phillip had lost his love of chips, which didn't surprise me. I even tested it by having a bag of chips at hand. I opened the bag, ate one, and offered some to him, only to see him politely refuse, and non-verbally communicate "no way!"

But there was something very surprising that happened that night. Donna, one of the women who was enrolled in the online version of the weight-loss program was watching me do the session on a live feed on her computer. Donna had been trying to give up chips for years without success. So while I was helping Phillip break up with chips, Donna was listening to the instructions I was giving Phillip and doing them herself. By the end of the session, Donna had lost the urge to eat chips.

I had no idea at the time that Donna was doing this. It wasn't until the following day when I received an email from her telling me that my Like to Dislike session had worked for her via the web. [Another person in the weight-loss group audience that night was also following along and had such a strong reaction that she had to leave the room because she felt like she might get sick.]

Not everybody notices the change right away. For example, I worked with one of our Amen Clinics staff members on her love of bagels. She used to eat one every morning and felt like she couldn't start her day without one. At the end of our session, she said it had minimal effect on her. Six months later, however, she has still not eaten any bagels.

How Does Like to Dislike Work?

To help you understand how this technique works, I'm going to take you through my own Like to Dislike session step-by-step. You will see how simple it is, and how successful it can be, especially when it is used by someone who has been adequately trained in NLP. When trying this on your own or in the hands of someone who doesn't have appropriate training, results can be inconsistent.

1. Are you ready and willing to make this change today?
Was I 100 percent committed to giving up sweet potato fries for the rest of my life? Yes, I had absolutely no hesitation about never eating sweet potato fries again.

If you have any hesitation, or if you aren't 100 percent ready and willing to give up the food, results can be inconsistent, and I suggest not doing it until you **are** *ready.*

2. What is the food you like and the food you greatly dislike?
The food I like is sweet potato fries, and feta cheese is the food I dislike.

Here, you want to think carefully about the foods you choose. This helpful technique works best if you choose something very specific. The more specific the better. Don't choose something that's too broad, such as "sugar" because sugar is in thousands of things, including brain healthy foods like fruit and low-fat yogurt—even unsweetened yogurt contains some natural sugars—and you may have a negative reaction to all of them. You may not even realize that sugar is contained in foods that you would like to continue eating, such as many store-bought salad dressings, spaghetti sauce, or ketchup.

I tell my patients that I want their choice to be "ecological," meaning in this context, that the food they choose isn't going to create problems in other areas for them.

Another reason why it's better to choose something specific is that you need to be able to have a mental image of the food. So with sugar, for example, you can't really get a mental image of thousands and thousands of products.

In addition, better results are typically achieved if you have a very strong negative *reaction to the food that you greatly dislike. For example, if a particular food or beverage turns your stomach, it's more likely that you'll have success.*

3. What does your mental image of the food you like look like?

My image of sweet potato fries is about one foot away from me at chest level. The image is in color as opposed to black and white. There is no frame around the image. The image is focused. The focus is steady. The image is still as opposed to moving. It is a bright image. It's important to note that I'm not "trying" to create this image. This is just what I see.

All of these qualities are called visual "submodalities." Ask yourself the following questions and write down your answers:

- *Where is the image located? How far away from you is it? At what level is it (are you looking up at it, down at it, to the left or right, etc.)?*
- *Is it in color or black and white?*
- *Is there a frame around the image?*
- *Is the image in focus?*
- *Is the focus steady or does it come in and out of focus?*
- *Is the image moving or still?*
- *How bright or dim is the image?*

4. What does your mental image of the food you like sound like?

There's a crunchy sound in my mouth. It's medium volume and it's an internal sound.

All of these qualities are called auditory "submodalities." Ask yourself the following questions and write down your answers:

- *Is there any sound associated with your mental image, and if so, what is the sound?*
- *Where is the sound located?*
- *How loud or soft is the sound?*
- *Where is the sound coming from—is it external or internal?*

5. What does your mental image of the food you like feel like?

It feels warm in my stomach. It has an intensity level of 7 out of 10. The shape of the feeling is the shape of my stomach, and the size of the feeling is the size of my stomach.

*All of these qualities are called kinesthetic or feeling "submodalities."
Ask yourself the following questions and write down your answers:*

- *Are there any feelings associated with your mental image, and if so, what are those feelings?*
- *What is the intensity level of the feeling on a scale of 1-10?*
- *What is the shape of the feeling?*
- *What is the size of the feeling?*

It may seem odd to associate a feeling with a food, but people give all kinds of different answers here. They may say they feel it in their heart, their chest, their hands, or anywhere. It doesn't have to make logical sense. Remember, we are dealing with the unconscious mind here.

6. Break state.
Here the practitioner told me to "think of the color green" as a way to "break state" and get away from my mental image of sweet potato fries.

There are many ways you can break state. For example, you can think of a color, recite the pledge of allegiance, say a prayer, or sing a song silently to yourself.

7. What does your mental image of the food you greatly dislike look like?
My image of feta cheese is about one foot away from me but about eight inches higher up. I have to look upwards at it toward my forehead. The image is in color even though feta cheese is white. It has a black frame around it. The image is focused and steady. The image is still as opposed to moving. It is a little bit dimmer than the image of the fries.

Ask yourself the same questions and write down your answers:

- *Where is the image located? How far away from you is it? At what level is it (are you looking up at it, down at it, to the left or right, etc.)?*
- *Is it in color or black and white?*
- *Is there a frame around the image?*
- *Is the image in focus?*

- *Is the focus steady or does it come in and out of focus?*
- *Is the image moving or still?*
- *How bright or dim is the image?*

8. What does your mental image of the food you greatly dislike sound like?
There's no sound.

Ask yourself the same questions and write down your answers:

- *Is there any sound associated with your mental image, and if so, what is the sound?*
- *Where is the sound located?*
- *How loud or soft is the sound?*
- *Where is the sound coming from—is it external or internal?*

9. What does your mental image of the food you greatly dislike feel like?
It feels disgusting on the roof of my mouth. It has an intensity level of 8 out of 10. The shape of the feeling is like little chunks in my mouth, and the size of the feeling is the size of my mouth.

Ask yourself the same questions and write down your answers:

- *Are there any feelings associated with your mental image, and if so, what are those feelings?*
- *What is the intensity level of the feeling on a scale of 1-10?*
- *What is the shape of the feeling?*
- *What is the size of the feeling?*

10. Break state.
Here, I broke state again to get away from my mental image of feta.

11. Now replace the visual qualities of the mental image of the food you like with the visual qualities of the mental image of the food you greatly dislike.
The #1 most important thing I did is move the location of the fries from being at chest level to above eye level where the feta was. The fries were

bright but the feta was dim so I envisioned turning a knob on a control panel to dim the image of the fries in my mind. The fries had no frame but the feta had a black frame, so I put a black frame around the fries.

Both of the images were in color, about one foot in front of me, focused, steady focus, and still so I didn't change any of that.

I like to think of this part of the process as if you were using a photo editing program that allows you to take a photo and increase or decrease brightness, change it to black and white, add or subtract a frame, crop it to make it look closer or farther away from you, and more.

It's very important to understand that you aren't replacing the image of sweet potato fries with the image of feta cheese. You are replacing the "qualities" of the image with the "qualities" of the other image.

12. Now replace the sound qualities of the mental image of the food you like with the sound qualities of the mental image of the food you greatly dislike.
I replace the crunchy sound of the fries with the absence of sound, which I had with the feta cheese.

13. Now replace the feeling qualities of the mental image of the food you like with the feeling qualities of the mental image of the food you greatly dislike.
I changed the warm feeling of the fries to have the feeling of disgust in my mouth I had with the feta cheese and changed the intensity level to 8 out of 10. I imagined myself chewing on the fries and feeling the shape of little chunks on the roof of my mouth, and changed the size of the feeling to the size of my mouth.

14. Now lock these changes into place.
I imagined closing a vault or a safe, turning the dial and scrambling the combination so it can't be opened again.

15. Break state.
I thought of a color.

16. Test it.

When the practitioner asked me how I felt about sweet potato fries, the mere thought of them made me feel very nauseated for about twenty minutes. For me, this was quite surprising because in my lifetime, I have only rarely ever felt nauseated.

At this point in the process, it is not uncommon for people to experience nausea when thinking about eating the food they used to like. In most cases, the feelings of nausea associated with the food subside over time. For example, when I see sweet potato fries now, I do not experience any sensation of nausea. I simply do not want to eat them.

However, if you have a very sensitive stomach or respond strongly to suggestion, I highly recommend that you work with a professional because the negative response can be very strong.

When I test how well the process has worked with my patients, I like to make it more dramatic by "magically" having a sample of the food available and putting it in front of them.

After I finish a session with someone, I sometimes point out something that usually takes them by surprise: the fact that throughout this entire process, we never talk about, think about, or change the way the food tastes. It's all about the mental image we have of the food.

The Problem Food I Like
Write down a specific food or drink you like, but want to avoid.

The Food I Greatly Dislike
Write down a food that you absolutely can't stand.

_____

_____

Can Like to Dislike Work For Me?

Success depends on your individual needs. Compared to some of the other therapeutic tools I use to help end emotional overeating, Like to Dislike is more like a "quick fix." It's best designed for people who just need help with one or two problem foods. It isn't designed to deal with the underlying emotions that drive you to eat in the first place.

For many of the emotional overeaters I work with, however, Like to Dislike is a powerful first step to reaching their goals. Seeing that you can *stop eating a trigger food can show you that you are actually capable of changing your behavior. And that belief in yourself can lead the way to more transformative changes that help you release the underlying emotions that are driving your overeating in the first place.*

In some cases, patients are so thrilled that they've made strides toward changing their behavior that they come back to me and ask for more help in conquering their negative emotions. For these emotional overeaters, I combine Like to Dislike with more intensive change work, including the techniques you will learn about in the following chapter.

Chapter 8

DISCONNECT THE BRIDGES FROM THE PAST

Learn From the Past Without Emotionally Reliving It

Many people overeat as a way to deal with past hurts or emotional traumas. Troubled childhoods, difficult parents, being abused, losing your job, going through a divorce—all of these stressful events can cause actual physical changes in the brain that lead to anxiety, depression, and emotional overeating. Whenever we experience trauma, it often gets stuck in our unconscious mind, even if it happened decades earlier, and it can hurt you.

Sharon's Brain SPECT Scan

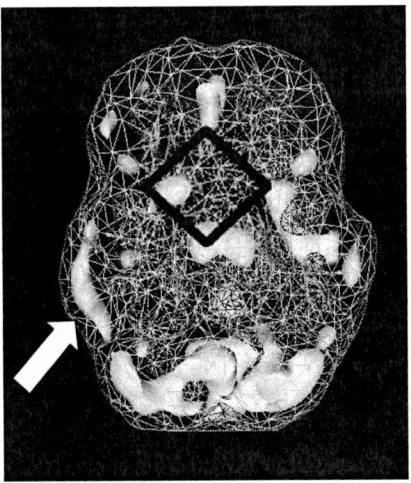

Sharon came to see me for being anxious and overweight. On her SPECT scan she had an emotional trauma pattern. We call it the "Diamond Plus pattern" because the emotional part of the brain is overactive in such a way that it looks like a diamond.

The Diamond Plus pattern shows areas of overactivity in the emotional parts of the brain.

- Top of the diamond is the anterior cingulate gyrus (people get stuck on negative thoughts)
- Middle points of the diamond are the basal ganglia (often associated with anxiety)
- Bottom of the diamond is the thalamo-limbic brain (often associated with sadness)
- Plus part of the diamond is the right temporal lobe (where people tend to relive and re-enact past experiences and also become hypervigilant reading the intentions of others)

When I first asked her about emotional trauma she said she'd never experienced any emotional trauma. I asked her five times, and each time she said there hadn't been any emotional trauma in her life.

I then asked her to tell me why she overate. "I don't know," she said, "Sometimes I just feel so nervous, and food makes me feel better, at least for a while."

One of the most effective tools I use with my patients is something I call "disconnecting the bridges from the past." Whenever you feel upset, write down how you feel in the moment, such as, "I feel really anxious," then go back in your mind to the first time in your life that you can remember having that feeling.

In Sharon's case, whenever she felt anxious she had trouble breathing. When I asked her what she felt, she said it felt like she was suffocating.

I asked her to go back in her mind to the first time in her life that she could remember having trouble breathing. Her mind immediately went back to a time when she was four years old and had a piece of steak stuck in her throat. She turned blue and thought she was going to die. She remembers someone from behind her squeezing her really hard and dislodging the piece of meat. She was so upset that she couldn't stop crying. Her parents gave her cake and ice cream to calm her down.

Once she understood the emotional bridge, she was able to disconnect her anxiety from the event and made significant progress on her anxiety and her weight over the next year. Learning how to deal with stress and disconnecting the traumas from the past are critical pieces to ending emotional overeating. If you have emotional trauma, don't run from it, make sure you get help for it.

My First Experience
Think back to the first time you experienced a bothersome emotion or emotions in the context of overeating, food, or your health, and write it down here. Becoming consciously aware of the event may help you begin to disconnect that emotion from the past.

_____

_____

_____

_____

_____

For some people, like Sharon, becoming consciously aware of how an emotion is tied to a past event is all it takes to begin the process of disconnecting the bridges from the past. For other people, however, conscious awareness isn't enough to free them from troublesome emotions. When that is the case, working with your unconscious mind can help. Larry uses a unique set of therapeutic tools that engage the unconscious mind to help you disconnect the bridges from the past. Here, he explains more about that.

"I Don't Know Why I'm Doing This…"

In the case study above, when Daniel asked Sharon why she overate, she said, "I don't know why." Typically, any time you say, "I don't know why I'm doing this, but…" it's telling you that it's your unconscious mind that's driving the behavior rather than your conscious mind. The good news is that we can figure out why you keep doing something that you consciously know isn't good for you, like overeating,

On the flip side, merely knowing why *you are doing something doesn't necessarily solve the problem. That can be the trouble with traditional therapy. In traditional therapy, you can talk about past traumas for years and still be unable to disconnect from the hurtful emotions that are driving your overeating. To quickly disconnect emotions tied to past events, it is critical to get your unconscious mind on board.*

Is there anything you do that you can't consciously explain? Eating before you go out to dinner? Waiting until everyone leaves your party then bingeing on leftovers? Eating in the middle of the night? Use the following chart to write them down.

I Don't Know Why I…

_____

_____

_____

_____

_____

Getting Your Unconscious Mind to Help You Disconnect From Negative Emotions

To help people disconnect from emotions tied to past events, I use a variety of techniques, including Time Empowerment Techniques®, which were created and developed by Dr. Tad James and his son, Dr. Matthew James, one of my personal teachers. They are a novel, relatively quick, and safe set of therapeutic techniques that help people release the negative emotions and limiting decisions associated with many different problems, including emotional overeating. In fact, I have personally used these techniques in helping people with various emotional problems such as depression, anger management, relationship issues, career stagnation, gambling and sex addictions, and various psychosomatic complaints, oftentimes curing the entire problem.

With this therapy, you go back to your earliest memory associated with a negative emotion, and then we work on disconnecting the emotions. To help you gain a better understanding of this therapy, I am going to share some of the most common questions my patients ask and how I answer them.

Why is it important to go back to that very first memory? *I like to say that your memories are like a string of pearls, with each pearl representing a significant emotional event. The string is the neurological circuitry that holds the pearls together. With this therapy, we're going back to that first pearl—the first event associated with the negative emotion. When you release that first pearl, the whole string of pearls falls apart. You are no longer able to access the inappropriate negative emotion.*

How does my unconscious mind go back to my earliest memory? *One of the first steps in this process is bringing the unconscious mind and the conscious mind into alliance with each other rather than working against each other. Then we can begin the change work and ask your unconscious mind about the first time you experienced a negative emotion.*

Although your conscious mind may pinpoint an experience when you were five, ten, or thirteen years old, your unconscious mind can remember even farther back in time than your conscious mind can comprehend. Often, my patients will say that their earliest unconscious memory associated with the negative emotion was at the time of birth or during infancy. It may not make any sense consciously, but that's okay. Once we have discovered that earliest memory, then we can work on disconnecting the negative emotions associated with it, which will cause the problem to disappear.

It worked for Joe. He had been carrying around deep-seated anger that fueled his overeating for forty years of his life. When we did our session, Joe's unconscious mind discovered the earliest memory of his anger and was able to release his negative feelings. Without the anger, Joe no longer felt the need to eat as a way to deal with those emotions. He was ecstatic to put an end to his emotional overeating and to the angry feelings that had been gnawing at him for decades.

Do I have to tell you about that painful first event? *With this type of therapy, you don't have to tell me what the painful event or memory was. You just need to have a mental image of it. Then we work on letting go of the inappropriate anger, sadness, fear, and guilt you associate with it. For example, I actually have no idea what was causing Joe's anger all those years, and I don't* need *to know. With most of my patients, I never know what that first experience was. This also significantly helps reduce the length of time needed to get results, by not spending valuable time "re-hashing one's story" session after session.*

What happens to my memories? *With this therapy, you don't "erase" the memory of painful events. You just shed the burdensome emotions associated with them that don't serve you in your life today. The memory is still there, but there's no emotion attached to it. It's more like data. You can acknowledge that it's there, but it doesn't bother you anymore.*

Is this like "recovered memory" therapy? *This therapy is* not *hypnosis, recovered memories, or regressive hypnotherapy. At no time am I* suggesting *where to go in your past or what to remember. I am* eliciting *your memories as opposed to* suggesting *or* installing *memories. This is a very important distinction.*

Do I have to relive my painful memories? *With this therapy, you never have to relive or rehash the painful events in your life. In Joe's case, he was happy to overcome his emotional overeating, but he was even more excited about the fact that he was able to do so* without *having to relive those painful experiences and emotions in my office.*

So much of traditional psychotherapy involves drudging up difficult experiences and emotions and reliving every gut-wrenching moment of them. With this therapeutic technique, however, you never have to relive those moments. You view that first experience from a distance so you don't become mired in the emotions.

This is so important for people who have suffered emotional trauma and don't want to have to go through the experience again in a therapy setting. In fact, some people avoid seeking help for past emotional traumas specifically because it's too painful to talk about it.

Is ending emotional overeating the only benefit? *Even if a patient comes to see me specifically for help with emotional overeating, the results can be much more far-reaching. Take my patient Kimberly, for example. More than 100 pounds overweight, Kimberly came to see me for emotional overeating.*

After we released the negative emotions she had been holding on to due to physical, verbal, emotional, and sexual abuse as a child and adolescent, she no longer felt the need to eat to cover up those emotions. And in addition, by removing those negative emotions, she found that her approach to her relationships was more positive and her attitude at work had improved. She was on the path to getting thinner, more loving, and more successful—all from one single session!

This is because there is some degree of overlap in various contexts of your life when you release anger, for example. Though the primary aim of this session was for help in emotional overeating, the anger she released created a neurological chain reaction into other parts of her life.

But, Doctor, don't I need fear? *Several patients have asked me if* *releasing emotions like fear could pose a problem. They have asked me, "Don't I need fear to protect myself?" When this is the case, I go over two important things:*

1. *First, I question them if fear is really "protecting" them. Isn't fear actually filling your body with chemicals that create tension in the body and have detrimental effects on your health? Isn't it actually your* knowledge, good judgment, *and* intelligence *that is protecting you by helping you make wise choices? The negative emotion of fear associated with a past event isn't serving a purpose anymore.*

2. *Second, I explain that even if I wanted to completely remove such a primal emotion, like fear, I couldn't do it. It is impossible. The primitive brain is wired to initiate the "fight-or-flight" response when appropriate, and no amount of this type of therapy will change that. For example, if you are hiking and come face-to-face with a mountain lion, you are still going to have the fight-or-flight response. The fear we are releasing with this therapy is the inappropriate fear you experience when that fight-or-flight response kicks into overdrive due to past emotional events and is no longer appropriate.*

What's a timeline? *To help my patients go back to their earliest memories, I have them take on a mental voyage on their timeline. What's a timeline? It's the unconscious orientation of your past and future. If I asked your unconscious mind right now to quickly point to your past without thinking about it, where would you point? If I asked you to point to your future, in which direction would you point?*

For some people, their past is behind them and their future is in front of them. For others, their past is to the left and their future is to the right. Still others may point to the ground as their past and up to the ceiling as their future. There is no right or wrong answer. But your timeline can be a helpful indicator of potential issues, such as if you are "stuck in the past," "struggling to get ahead," or having trouble being present in the moment.

For example, my patient Kristy came to see me for career and relationship problems. She told me it felt like she was always fighting an uphill battle trying to get ahead at work and with her boyfriend. When I elicited her timeline, she indicated by pointing that her past was down to the ground behind her, and that her future was up ahead of her. If you connected those two points, they formed a steep angle—she really was going uphill!

Together, we worked on re-orienting her timeline so her future wasn't a steep hill any longer and that she was comfortable in making this change. As she walked out of our session, she told me she felt like she was literally gliding on air into her future. At her follow-up appointment a month later she told me that this was a profound shift for her, and that life was no longer always an uphill battle.

Besides discovering my earliest memory, what can I learn from my timeline? *The benefits of mentally traveling back into your past go beyond just discovering what your earliest memory was; they also include understanding the lessons that needed to be learned from that experience. When you experience an event at a very young age, you experience it from a certain perspective. Through this technique, you can view the same event now from a different perspective. By doing so, you may be able to see, hear, or feel something that you weren't able to when the event first occurred. You can then bring this new knowledge back with you to the present moment allowing you to retain any positive learnings from the event.*

Is there anything else I can gain from this type of therapy? *There's a lot more to Time Empowerment Techniques® than what you see here in this chapter. In sessions, I am cooperatively guiding my patients along their timeline into their past, into their future, and back to the present. This therapy can be used to help you install goals into your future to help keep you on track with your healthy eating plan, eliminate anxiety surrounding an event such as an upcoming family dinner or eating engagement, re-orient your timeline if necessary, and much more. These are advanced techniques that are best performed with the aid of a Master Practitioner of Time Empowerment Techniques®.*

How Donna Let Go of Negative Emotions

Remember Donna, the woman who watched me do a Like to Dislike session online and stopped eating chips? After having success in kicking her chips habit, she came to see me for additional help with her emotional overeating. Chips, she had realized, wasn't her only problem.

Every time Donna went to social functions or parties, she felt compelled to have a drink in her hand at all times and to gobble up any available finger foods. Donna believed that she was suffering from what psychiatrists call "social anxiety." I sometimes question the diagnoses given to people by previous doctors because though they often 'fit' the 'standard' DSM-4-TR diagnostic criteria, they also tend to lock a person into a category, which often in psychiatry has no real "cure." Then, that person's outcome will depend on medications and 'talking' about their problem. However, by using highly specialized techniques, "social anxiety" can disappear or greatly diminish. What was previously deemed non-curable can many times be essentially eliminated if the problem is tied to negative emotions from the past.

With Donna, she wasn't nervous about anyone who was attending these events so she couldn't understand why she felt so on edge.

In our session, she went back to the first time she felt that way. It was when she was a child and living in a home with parents who were verbally and emotionally abusive. Donna never knew what to expect when she was at home, whether her parents were going to be loving or whether they were going to fly off the handle. To protect herself, she learned to be hypervigilant around other people. Hypervigilance is a state of being in which you are "on high alert" at all times, ready to deal with any suspected threats.

Donna was on high alert at social gatherings, and she ate to comfort herself. She had never made the link between the way her parents had treated her as a child and her actions today. "So that's *why I'm doing that," she said.*

The hypervigilance may have served a purpose when she was a child, but there was no need for it now. Nobody at these events was going to be abusive to her. This emotion was unnecessary and creating other problems for her, including overeating to "cope with her social anxiety problem."

Discovering that this was where her problem stemmed from was only part of the process. It wasn't enough to help her overcome the hypervigilance she felt at social events. Together using Time Empowerment Techniques®, we released her hypervigilance, and she can now go to parties without spending the entire time grazing at the buffet table.

Months after our session, Donna contacted me to let me know that she had since attended several wedding receptions and a Thanksgiving dinner. She was thrilled that she didn't feel anxious or hypervigilant and had absolutely no compulsion to gobble up hors d'oeuvres or have a drink in her hand. She was able to feel relaxed and be herself, and she proudly socialized with people fearlessly.

In one or two sessions, Donna's "social anxiety" was gone. My guess is that if you asked most traditional psychiatrists if it's possible to get rid of social anxiety in a few sessions without medications, they would say "absolutely not." But when you work with someone highly trained, recruit your unconscious mind into the process, and release the negative emotions associated with your earliest memory, it is possible.

How Charlie Shifted His Values

This brings me back to your values and motivators, which we wrote about in chapter 3. Most of the people with emotional overeating issues who come to see me are filled with negative motivators, the motivators that set you up for a lifetime of yo-yo dieting. But after we disconnect the negative emotions associated with the past and sometimes re-orient the timeline, those values and motivators can shift dramatically so they will keep you on track for the rest of your life.

Remember Charlie, the patient I wrote about in chapter 3? He was the 350-pound man who wanted to stop eating butter and whose list of values included nothing but negative motivators. After we did this therapy, he came up with a completely different list of values with positive motivators. The change made such a difference in his life, he wrote me a letter and gave me permission to share it with others. Here is an excerpt:

> Dr. Momaya,
>
> I wanted to take a moment to thank you for your incredible insights and assistance. I must admit to initially being highly skeptical of your methods and results. My original intention was actually more exploratory than results directed. Yet, I found you up to my challenges and more than willing to help. Not to mention that turning off the butter craving is still in effect months later.
>
> I especially was impacted by your work in assisting me in understanding the root causes of my weight-management issues. The first session where we addressed "why" issues and particularly the fact that so much of my response was moving "away from" things but not "toward what I really desired," spurred me to focus on being more proactive toward what I wanted.
>
> The extended therapy was so beneficial in addressing emotions that I never would have believed existed or were there in my subconscious. I must admit it was not an easy session but I believe it has made a profound difference in my understanding of self and in my desire to move toward the things I want, like health. And, as the business cut-to-the-chase guy I am, it was efficient and effective.
>
> Finally, the revisiting of my original goals and the way that they had changed due to the sessions was nothing short of amazing to me. I am still working through my new SMART goals and trying to comprehend the other concepts you shared with me. But, I know I am on the right track for long-term success in my health

management because I am moving towards what I want, not away from all the stuff I have dealt with over the years. My new weight loss project is coming along and in about twelve months I should be where I intend. All this is due to your professional care along with your sense of personal commitment and challenge.

Thank you,
Charlie

Overcoming Skepticism

Some people are understandably skeptical about the idea of recruiting the unconscious mind to help release negative emotions. I understand that it is a new concept that can be difficult for some people to grasp at first.

Tony is a prime example. He made an appointment with me after seeing an article Daniel wrote about me and my work with emotional overeaters in his weekly Brain in the News *email newsletter.*

Tony came into my office and before we even began to talk about why he was there, he said he wasn't sure about all this "unconscious mind stuff" and asked if I had any referrals. Of course, I told him, and I offered him testimonials from several patients who have given me permission to share their experiences, like Charlie did in his letter above.

That helped Tony feel more confident about our session, and he relaxed and began to open up. Interestingly enough, as we worked on his negative emotions, I could visibly see that the process was working. I noticed that with each negative emotion that was released, Tony would gradually swing his crossed leg. He was completely unaware of it. The leg swing was an ideomotor signal to me that the release work was working.

Getting Your Unconscious Mind and Conscious Mind to Work Together

After our session, Tony was convinced. He said he felt freer than ever and more confident that he would be able to lose weight and keep it off. At this point, I let him know that the important change work we had just done was only part *of the solution to his weight problem. We had gotten his unconscious mind on board, but we needed to make sure he had the conscious know-how to follow through on his plan to lose weight.*

I told Tony it was his job now to take action and stay focused outside my office. That's where Daniel's book The Amen Solution *and brain health comes in. Your conscious mind must know what to do to achieve a healthy weight, and you must optimize your brain to help you stay on track. When Tony got both his unconscious and conscious mind working together, he finally began to shed the weight he'd been carrying around for so many years.*

Chapter 9

TAME YOUR INNER CHILD

Learn to Say "No" to Yourself and Others

Do you have a war going on inside your head? Most emotional overeaters do. Perhaps the following inner dialogue will sound familiar to you.

> *"I had such a crummy day, I need some chocolate."*
>
> *"But I shouldn't have chocolate because I'm trying to lose weight."*
>
> *"But I want it, and it tastes so good, and it makes me feel so good. And I had such a rotten day."*
>
> *"But it makes me fat, and I hate being fat."*
>
> *"But it's just a little chocolate. I ate a really healthy lunch and dinner. I deserve to have something yummy."*
>
> *"But I have to get out of this habit of eating it whenever I feel bad."*
>
> *"Maybe I'll just have one square. That's not so bad."*
>
> *"Hmmm… just one square? Yeah, that's not so bad. Research even shows that eating some dark chocolate is good for you."*
>
> *"Right, so I'm just going to have one square."*
>
> *"Yeah, one square. Okay."*

"Wow, that one square was really good, but it wasn't enough. Now I need another one."

"I know I shouldn't, but it was really good, wasn't it? Okay, just one or two more."

"Well, now that I ate that much, I may as well eat the whole bar."

"Ugh… I shouldn't have eaten that entire bar of chocolate. I feel gross now, and I feel like a failure. I'm doomed to be fat for the rest of my life. Why can't I just say "no?"

All of the information in this program is designed to help you win the war in your head between the adult, thoughtful part of your brain that knows what you should do and your pleasure centers, which are run by a spoiled, demanding inner child who *always* wants what he or she wants *whenever* he or she wants it.

Your pleasure centers are always looking for a good time:

- They *crave* the ice cream.
- They *want* the double cheeseburgers.
- They *urge* you to drive for miles and stand in line for the fresh cinnamon rolls.
- They *focus* on having the second piece of cake.

Left unchecked, your inner child is often whispering to you like a naughty little friend:

- Eat it now…
- It's okay…
- We deserve it…
- Come on, let's have some fun…
- Don't be so uptight…
- Live a little….
- We already had one bowl of ice cream, just one more won't hurt…

- We'll be better tomorrow... I promise.

Without adult supervision, your inner child lives only in the moment, and he or she can ruin your life.

Strengthen Your Prefrontal Cortex

To balance your pleasure centers and tame your inner child, there is an area in the front part of your brain called the prefrontal cortex (PFC), which helps you think about what you do before you do it. The prefrontal cortex is called the executive part of the brain because it acts like the boss at work and is involved with judgment, forethought, planning, and self-control. It thinks about your future, not just about what you want in the moment.

Instead of thinking about the chocolate cake, it is the rational voice in your head that says:

- I need to *avoid* having a big belly.
- I'm getting *concerned* about my bulging medical bills.
- When I say, "No," I mean it.

It is your prefrontal cortex that is reading and doing the exercises in this program while your inner child keeps telling you, "Put the program down. Don't trust these guys. They'll ruin all our fun."

When your PFC is strong, it reins in your inner child, so that you can have fun, but in a thoughtful, measured way. To put a stop to emotional overeating, it is critical to strengthen your PFC and put your inner child into time-out whenever he or she acts up. Even if you have done some of the change work detailed in this program, it is still very important to strengthen your PFC.

It is also critical to watch your internal dialogue and be a good parent to yourself, not one who is abusive or mean. I have taught parenting classes for many years, and the two words that embody good parenting, even for your inner child, are *firm* and *kind*. When you make a mistake with food or with your health, look for ways to learn from your mistakes, but always in a loving way.

To make it easier to say "no" to your inner child, you must strengthen your prefrontal cortex. Here's how you do that.

Avoid things that lower activity in the prefrontal cortex:

- Diets high in refined carbohydrates (crackers, white bread, cookies, pretzels, etc.)
- Alcohol
- Excessive caffeine
- Sugar—check nutrition labels for hidden sugars
- Stress—use the stress-relieving exercises in Chapter 5

Do the things that boost activity in the prefrontal cortex:

- Do at least 30 minutes of exercise every day.
- Meditate daily—see Chapter 5.
- Set goals by completing the One-Page Miracle exercise from Chapter 3.
- Enlist others you trust to provide outside supervision so when you're having trouble saying "no," they can say it for you.
- Practice willpower by saying "no" to your inner child.
- From a supplement standpoint, green tea, rhodiola, and L-tyrosine are helpful.

Say "No" to the Food Pushers

Your inner child isn't the only one who will tempt you to stray from your healthy eating habits. Food pushers are all around us. When I became a grandfather for the first time, I couldn't wait to visit my new grandson, Elias. When I went to my daughter's home, a friend of mine was also visiting. She asked me if I wanted something to eat, and I said no, I wasn't hungry. A few minutes later, she asked me again, and I told her no again. I thought that would be the end of that discussion, but she continued to ask me an additional five times if I wanted something to eat!

I call these people food pushers. And as you embark on your journey to end emotional overeating, you need to be aware that on a daily basis, you will face many types of food pushers who will try to derail your efforts.

Sometimes, it's the people we love the most who push the most food our way. When you feel down or stressed, they offer you a cookie or a chocolate bar to make you feel better. When you get that promotion, they celebrate it with cake and ice cream.

Plus, as I like to say, you are who you eat with. We tend to adopt the habits of those around us. If you surround yourself with people who are overeaters, it is easy to get sucked into their habits.

Sometimes, the people you love may willfully try to undermine your efforts. When you start eating in a healthy way and losing weight, it can make those around you uncomfortable, especially if they are overweight or have their own issues with emotional overeating. Deep down, some people—even those who love you the most—don't want you to succeed because it will make them feel like more of a failure.

For others, their habits are so ingrained that they simply don't know how to react to your new lifestyle. Many of my patients notice this kind of behavior with their families, friends, and coworkers. For example, your mother might bake a cake for your birthday even though you told her you are trying to curb your sugar intake. At work, the receptionist may continue to bring in doughnuts and coffee for your morning meetings because she thinks she's being "nice." Or, when you're hosting your church group's weekly Bible study, members might show up with a box of cupcakes or a loaf of banana bread because they feel bad showing up empty-handed even though you specifically asked them *not* to bring anything.

On the flip side, your new eating habits may rub off on your friends and family. When people see the new and improved you, they may be inspired to get on the brain healthy bandwagon.

The people around you can either hurt or help your chances for success. This is why it is so important to encourage the people in your social network to get on board with your healthy eating habits.

When you enlist your friends, family, and coworkers to support you in your efforts to eat in a healthy way, it is less likely that they will push food on you. It is also critical to create a strong support group of like-minded brain healthy role models, such as our online community, where you can turn for help when you need it.

Food Pushers are Everywhere

Almost everywhere you go during your daily life, you will see reminders of the foods you used to crave or that you ate mindlessly. Drive to work, and you'll have to pass by the fast-food place where you used to order three cheeseburgers, jumbo fries, and an all-you-can-drink soda. Take a cruise to Alaska because you want to see the beautiful scenery, and you'll have to face unbelievably copious amounts of food and desserts at the buffet not to mention the free-flowing alcohol.

Even though churches can be good for your soul, many of them can be terrible for your waistline. I have gone to church my whole life and lately have been frustrated by the poor food they serve their parishioners.

Recently, I went to church near my home. My wife Tana dropped our daughter off at children's church, and I went to get us our seats. As I walked in, I passed by boxes of doughnuts for sale at $1 a piece, I saw men cooking sausage and bacon, and I saw hundreds of hot dog buns stacked up for after the service.

I was so irritated that when my wife joined me she saw me making notes to myself on my phone. She gave me one of those disapproving looks that only she can give me about typing on my phone in church. Then I showed her what I had typed in: "Go to church and get dollar doughnuts, sausage, bacon, hot dogs ... send people to heaven early. They need to know how to become a brain healthy church."

Tana agreed and forgave my indiscretion. Work to help your church, school, business, and family become brain healthy.

Who are the food pushers in your life? It is important to identify the food pushers you face in your daily life. Write them down here.

My Food Pushers
Write down the people, places, and things that tempt you to overeat. This could be a long list, so use an extra sheet of paper if you need to.

_____

_____

_____

_____

_____

Tips for Dealing With Food Pushers

Learning to deal with and say "no" to all of these pushers in the home, on the town, at work, at school, and at church is critical to your success. It's up to you to let your loved ones know that you've changed and you don't want to comfort yourself or celebrate your successes with foods that are making you fat and miserable. If you have done some of the change work involving the unconscious mind that is described in this book, it will be easier for you to say "no."

Here are some practical tips to help you fight back.

1. If you are going to a dinner with friends or family, call ahead to inform the host that you are on a special brain healthy diet and won't be able to eat certain foods. You only have to do this once

or twice before your friends start to ask you what they could serve that is brain healthy.

2. When going to parties, consider eating something at home first so you won't be hungry at the event.

3. Be upfront with food pushers. Explain that you are trying to eat a more balanced diet, and that when they offer you cake, chips, or pizza, it makes it more difficult for you.

4. Instead of going out to lunch or dinner with friends, choose activities that aren't centered around food, such as going for a walk.

5. When people offer seconds, tell them you are pleasantly full. If they insist, explain that you are trying to watch your calories. If they continue to push extra helpings on you, gently ask them why they are bent on sabotaging your efforts to be healthy.

6. Eat very slowly so when the host starts asking guests if they want seconds, you can say you are still working on your first helping. By the time you have finished, the second round of eating could be over, and you won't have to be subjected to the offer for more. See Chapter 6 for more on mindful eating.

7. Commit to taking control of your own body and don't let other people make you fat and stupid.

8. Tell restaurant servers "no bread" or "no chips" before you're seated.

9. Tell restaurant servers "no dessert" before they have a chance to bring the dessert tray to your table.

10. Inform parents and in-laws ahead of time that you won't be partaking in certain foods at family gatherings.

11. If the neighbor brings you a plate of chocolate chip cookies,

immediately "regift" them to someone else.

12. When a coworker suggests celebrating birthdays with cupcakes, recommend a healthy alternative.

13. Make a list of healthy meal and snack options and give it to your office administrator or church leaders.

14. Ask office administrators to get rid of the vending machines filled with sodas and candy.

15. At church, skip the doughnuts and coffee after the service and stand outside if you want to socialize.

16. At all-you-can-eat buffets, go for the salad (dressing on the side), steamed vegetables, and lean protein first, then after you have eaten that, go back if you're still hungry and want to try a higher-calorie item. Chances are you will eat a much smaller portion than if you had started with the fatty fare.

17. Bring your own healthy snacks to the movies so you don't have to go near the concession stand.

18. If you're at a sporting event, be aware that many ballparks and sports arenas are offering healthier options.

19. When temptation wins out, use the three-bite rule. Take three bites of the item, then toss it.

20. Donate money to the Girl Scouts rather than buying cookies.

21. When your spouse asks you to finish off the small amount of food left over from dinner, say "no," box it up, and put it in the refrigerator for another meal.

22. When it's your turn to host a party, send the leftovers home with your guests so you won't be tempted to eat them.

23. If someone in your dining party orders fries for the table, make sure you have a glass of water or green tea to sip on while they munch. It will keep you occupied and help prevent you from reaching for a fry, or two, or twenty.

24. At the grocery store checkout stand, keep your eyes focused on the checker so you don't have to look at the candy and other impulse-buy items calling out to you.

25. Make it a rule to *never* take free food samples *anywhere*!

My Say "No" to Food Pushers Strategies
*Write a list of strategies you will use to help you say
"no" to the food pushers.*

_____

_____

_____

_____

_____

_____

_____

_____

_____

These tips are all in line with a very important concept that Larry emphasizes with his patients.

I like the tips above because they illustrate the concept of "Personal Empowerment," which is something I work on with my patients. By Personal Empowerment, I mean being "at cause" for the things that happen in your life rather than being "the effect" of what happens in your life.

Do you see the difference? It may seem subtle to you, but it can make a huge difference in your life.

Being "at cause" means that you are "response-able" for your results. Being "the effect" means that you avoid taking "response-ability" for what is occurring, or has occurred, in your life: that it's because the waiter offered you free soda refills or your mother baked you a birthday cake that you are overweight and unhappy. When you are "the effect," it's as though you have no role in what is happening in your life.

Remember the "Blame ANT" that was introduced to you in Chapter 4? If you have a lot of Blame ANTs, you are likely living as "the effect."

With my patients, I help them notice the patterns in their life to help them understand if they are "at cause" or "the effect." If they are "the effect," I prod them to come up with answers about what their role has been in how they got to where they are now. I help them learn from that so they can begin being "at cause" for what happens in their life.

When you are "at cause," you are in control of your life rather than being controlled by outside forces. Knowing that you are "at cause" also gives you a sense of personal empowerment that helps you say "no" to the food pushers around you. I use this model when working with people with emotional issues, relationship issues, and much more.

The Three Circles: Know When You're Safe, Vulnerable, or in Danger

It is absolutely critical that you know what helps keep you on track with healthy eating, what makes you more likely to fall back into your old ways, and what puts you in imminent danger of overeating. To help my patients understand the people, places, and things that are helping them reach their goals and those that are putting them at greater risk for emotional overeating, I use an exercise called the Three Circles.

In the green circle, write down all the things that help you stay on track with your healthy eating. In the yellow circle, put things that make you more vulnerable for emotional overeating. In the red circle, list your danger zones—the things that put you in imminent danger of emotional overeating. Keep this page with you to help remind you what's helping you reach your goals and what is putting you at risk.

The following is an example from my patient Sarah, an emotional overeater who had issues with anxiety, depression, and road rage.

SARAH'S THREE CIRCLES

Green Circle

Meditating and praying daily
Doing deep breathing when I feel stress
Exercising at least 4 times a week
Correcting my negative thoughts
Looking at my One-Page Miracle every morning
Getting 7-8 hours of sleep
Listening to relaxing music
Taking my supplements
Eating mindfully

Skipping breakfast
Skipping exercise
Not getting enough sleep
Drinking alcohol
Dwelling on my mother's illness
Taking on too many projects
Focusing on the negative
Not taking my supplements
Sitting in traffic without my music
Not eating at the dining table

Being unable to meet a deadline at work
Arguing with my spouse
Not visiting my mother in the hospital
Having a road rage incident
Believing my negative thoughts
Eating while watching TV

Yellow Circle   **Red Circle**

MY THREE CIRCLES

Green Circle
*In this circle, write what helps keep
you safe and on track with your healthy eating.*

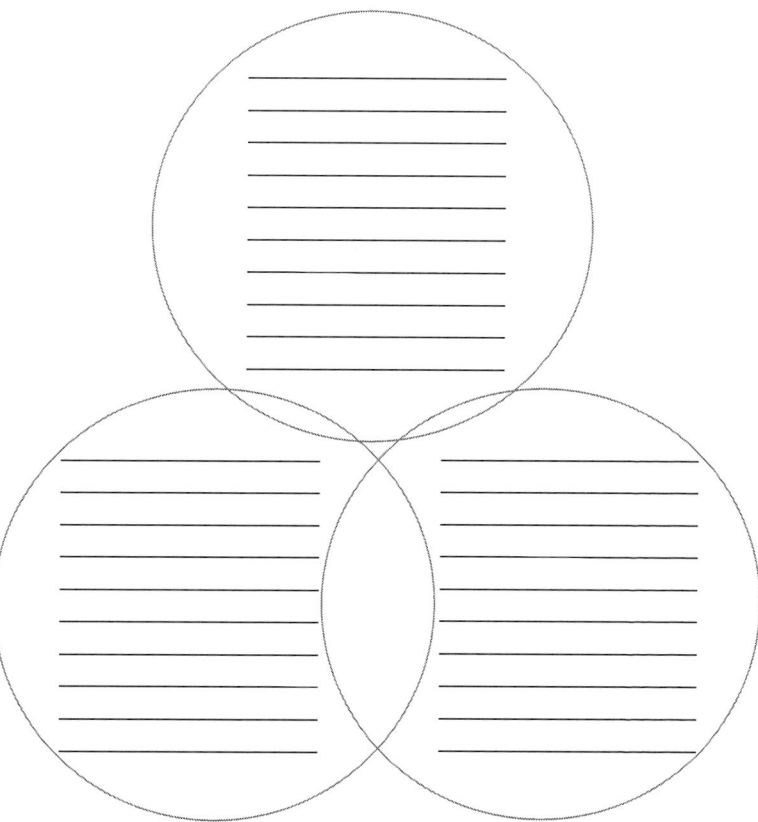

Yellow Circle
*In this circle, write what
makes you more vulnerable to
emotional overeating.*

Red Circle
*In this circle, write what puts
you in immediate danger of
emotional overeating.*

Chapter 10

EMERGENCY RESCUE FOR SETBACKS

Tips to Help You Stay on Track

The road to freedom from emotional eating is not a straight path. There can be many twists and turns along the way that steer you off course. Major life events, such as getting laid off, getting divorced, or losing a loved one can fire up the emotional centers of your brain and rekindle the urge to overeat. This is less likely to occur if you have done change work involving your unconscious mind, but it can still happen. Do not feel like you're a failure if you experience setbacks. The important thing is to acknowledge that you've had a setback and then get right back on the path of wellness.

To help my patients keep emotional overeating in check, I tell them to "H-A-L-T." H-A-L-T is an acronym that is commonly used in addiction treatment programs, but I find that it is also particularly helpful for emotional overeaters who have trouble coping with daily stress. H-A-L-T has proven to be a very effective way to keep people on track when they are trying to change their habits.

H-A-L-T stands for:

>Don't get too **H**ungry.

>Don't get too **A**ngry.

>Don't get too **L**onely.

>Don't get too **T**ired.

Don't Get Too Hungry

Going too long without food lowers your blood sugar levels, which can lead to a variety of emotional issues, including feelings of anxiety and irritability. These may be the very emotions that trigger your overeating.

Low blood sugar levels are also associated with lower overall brain activity, which is linked to an increase in cravings and impulsivity. Heightened anxiety and irritability coupled with more intense cravings and impulsivity is a recipe for emotional overeating. Keeping your blood sugar levels even throughout the day is critical to keep you on track.

Here are some tips to keep your blood sugar levels from getting too low.

- Eat a healthy breakfast—people who maintain weight loss eat a nutritious breakfast.

- Have smaller meals throughout the day. Eating big meals spikes your blood sugar levels then causes them to crash later on.

- Stay away from simple sugars and refined carbohydrates, such as candy, sodas, cookies, crackers, white rice, and white bread. These also spike your blood sugar then cause it to crash later on.

- The supplements alpha-lipoic acid and chromium have very good scientific evidence that they help balance blood sugar levels and can help with cravings.

My Don't Get Too Hungry Plan

Write down the things you plan to do to help prevent you from getting too hungry. Keep this list with you at all times.

_____

_____

_____

_____

_____

_____

Don't Get Too Angry

Uncontrolled anger can send you running to the cookie jar to calm your emotions. Here are some tips to help keep anger under control.

- When you feel mad, write down your thoughts and ask yourself, "Is it true?"

- Practice deep-breathing exercises. Use the deep-breathing exercises in Chapter 5.

- Meditate. Just a few minutes of meditation can help you refocus your thinking.

- Count to ten. When you get angry, count to ten before reaching for something to eat. Sometimes that short delay can be enough to calm your temper and interrupt the urge to eat.

- Get moving. If you feel anger bubbling up inside you, go for a walk or a short burst of exercise. This releases brain chemicals that help calm you down.

- Express your feelings. After you have calmed down, express your feelings in a non-confrontational way. Letting your anger fester can drive you to overeat.

My Don't Get Too Angry Plan

Write down the things you plan to do to help prevent you from getting too angry. Keep this list with you at all times.

_____

_____

_____

_____

_____

_____

Don't Get Too Lonely

Social skills and a positive social network are critical to your emotional well-being. Working on your current social situation is important to healing. Here are some tips to increase your social bonding.

- Enlist a team of supporters and healthy role models.

- Volunteer in your community.

- Join a church group, recreational sporting team, book group, or any other type of group that appeals to you.

- Make it a priority to spend time with your friends and family.

- Make a list of people you can reach out to when you are feeling sad, anxious, mad, or frustrated.

My Don't Get Too Lonely Plan

Write down the things you plan to do to help prevent you from getting too lonely. Keep this list with you at all times.

_____

_____

_____

_____

_____

_____

Don't Get Too Tired

A 2007 study found that sleep deprivation caused the emotional centers of the brain to become 60 percent more reactive to negative emotional stimuli. That means your brain simply can't cope as well with stressful situations, leading to worse moods, more anxiety, greater irritability, increased anger, and more frustration. And when your emotions are running wild, you are more apt to run to the refrigerator for solace.

In addition, lack of sleep lowers overall brain function, which leads to more bad decisions. Several studies have shown that lack of sleep leads to higher calorie intake and higher consumption of refined carbohydrates, which as you learned in the Don't Get Too Hungry section, causes blood sugar levels to spike and then crash.

If you routinely have trouble sleeping, I suggest keeping a sleep journal for at least a few weeks. Make copies of the following chart to track your sleep. It can help you pinpoint everyday habits that might be contributing to the problem.

MY SLEEP JOURNAL

Day/Date _____

Answer the following questions in the morning.
Last night, my bedtime ritual included: _____
(List things like a warm bath, meditation, reading, etc.)

Last night I went to bed at: _____ pm/am

Last night I fell asleep in: _____ minutes

Last night, I woke up: _____ times

During those times, I was awake for: _____ minutes

Last night, I got out of bed: _____ times

Things that disturbed my sleep: _____
(List any physical, mental, emotional, or environmental factors that affected your sleep.)

I slept for a total of: _____ minutes

I got out of bed this morning at: _____ am/pm

Upon waking, I felt: ___ refreshed ___ groggy ___ exhausted

Answer the following questions at night.
During the day, I fell asleep or napped: _____ times

During my naps, I slept for: _____ minutes

During the day, I felt: ___ refreshed ___ groggy ___ exhausted

My caffeine consumption: _____ amount _____ time of day

Medications or sleep aids I took: _____

Make sleep a priority to boost brain function, moods, and energy levels, and to improve judgment and self-control. Here are ten ways to make it easier to drift off to dreamland and get a good night's sleep. Remember that we are all unique individuals and what works for one person may not work for another. Keep trying new techniques until you find something that works.

- Maintain a regular sleep schedule—going to bed at the same time each night and waking up at the same time each day, including on weekends. Get up at the same time each day regardless of sleep duration the previous night.

- Create a soothing nighttime routine that encourages sleep. A warm bath, meditation, or massage can help you relax.

- Some people like to read themselves to sleep. If you are reading, make sure it isn't an action-packed thriller or a horror story—they aren't likely to help you drift off to sleep.

- Don't take naps! This is one of the biggest mistakes you can make if you have insomnia. Taking naps when you feel sleepy during the day compounds the nighttime sleep cycle disruption.

- Sound therapy can induce a very peaceful mood and lull you to sleep. Consider soothing nature sounds, soft music, wind chimes, or even a fan.

- Drink a mixture of warm milk, a teaspoon of vanilla (the real stuff, not imitation), and a few drops of stevia. This increases serotonin in your brain and helps you sleep.

- Take computers, video games, and cell phones out of the bedroom and turn them off an hour or two before bedtime to allow time to "unwind."

- Don't eat for at least two to three hours before going to bed.

- Regular exercise is very beneficial for insomnia, but don't do it within four hours of the time you hit the sack. Vigorous exercise late in the evening may energize you and keep you awake.

- Don't drink any caffeinated beverages in the late afternoon or evening. Also avoid chocolate, nicotine, and alcohol—especially at night. Although alcohol can initially make you feel sleepy, it interrupts sleep.

My Don't Get Too Tired Plan
Write down the things you plan to do to help prevent you from getting too tired. Keep this list with you at all times.

_____

_____

_____

_____

_____

_____

Remember That Your Emotional Health is a Work in Progress

Our emotions, like our bodies and lives, are in a constant state of change. Marriages, divorces, job transfers, pregnancies, injuries, illnesses, and hormonal transitions are just some of the many things that keep us in flux and that fire up our emotions.

We would like to emphasize again that the goal of this program is not to eliminate emotions completely from your life. Emotions play an important role in our lives and well-being. This program is designed to help you release any irrational, unnecessary, or inappropriate emotions and to learn to cope in more healthy ways with your day-to-day emotions. When you use the tools in this program, you can win the war with your emotions so you can feel at peace and end emotional overeating NOW.

ACKNOWLEDGMENTS

I am grateful to the myriad of people who have been instrumental in making *End Emotional Overeating NOW* a reality, especially all of the patients and professionals who have taught me so much about how the brain relates to the health of our bodies and minds. I am thankful to have had the opportunity to work on this program with Larry, who impressed me so much as a psychiatry intern that I hired him to join the Amen Clinics family. He continues to impress me today, and it has been a thrill for me to watch his unique and powerful approach to helping his patients take shape. I am especially grateful to my writing partner Frances Sharpe who was invaluable in the process of designing and completing this book. She remains committed to our mission and is a very thoughtful, hardworking, talented woman. Also, Dr. Kristen Willeumier, our Director of Research at the Amen Clinics, was a wonderful resource for research, collaboration, and encouragement. And, to Tana, my wife, my joy, and best friend, who is always ready to listen and give great suggestions and feedback. I love all of you. — *Daniel*

My deepest Gratitude goes to all of the diverse people who have, and continue to teach me about the Body/Mind/Spirit: Dr. Daniel Amen for giving me opportunities like this one, and having faith in me since the day I first met him as a Psychiatry Intern 10 years ago; Frances Sharpe for her enthusiasm in helping transcribe the concepts and ideas in my head beautifully into written word; Dr. Matthew James for his excellence in teaching me tools and techniques to do superb Change work for people; Byron Katie for helping me truly see myself and others without their 'story;' all of my patients and people I have worked with for their resilience, trust, and strength; my parents and sister for their unconditional and continuous love and support in every endeavor; and finally my Unconscious Mind, for its Source of Creativity, Energy Production, Learning States, and Alliance with my Conscious Mind and Higher Self. ~Love Always~ Love All Ways~ — *Larry*

ABOUT THE AUTHORS

Daniel G. Amen, M.D.

Daniel G. Amen, M.D., is a physician, child and adult psychiatrist, brain imaging specialist, and *New York Times* bestselling author. He is the writer, producer, and host of four highly successful public television programs, raising more than $20 million for public television. He is a Distinguished Fellow of the American Psychiatric Association and the CEO and medical director of Amen Clinics in Newport Beach and Fairfield, California; Bellevue, Washington; and Reston, Virginia.

Amen Clinics is the world leader in applying brain imaging science to everyday clinical practice and has the world's largest database of functional scans related to behavior, now totaling more than 60,000.

Dr. Amen is the author of thirty-five professional scientific articles and twenty-four books, including the *New York Times* bestsellers, *Change Your Brain, Change Your Body; Change Your Brain, Change Your Life;* and *Magnificent Mind at Any Age*. He is also the author of *Healing ADD, Healing the Hardware of the Soul, Making a Good Brain Great, The Brain in Love*, and the co-author of *Healing Anxiety and Depression* and *Preventing Alzheimer's*.

Dr. Amen spearheads the groundbreaking Amen Clinics retired NFL player brain imaging study and is intimately involved with The Daniel Challenge, a project of Pastor Rick Warren and Saddleback Church to create brain healthy churches.

Dr. Amen has appeared on the *Dr. Oz Show*, the *Today* show, *Good Morning America*, *The View*, *The Rachael Ray Show*, Larry King, *The Early Show*, CNN, HBO, Discovery Channel, and many other national television and radio programs. His national public television shows include *Change Your Brain, Change Your Life*; *Magnificent Mind at Any Age*; *The Brain in Love*; and *Change Your Brain, Change Your Body*.

A small sample of the organizations Dr. Amen has spoken for include the National Security Agency, the National Science Foundation, Harvard's Learning and the Brain Conference, The Million Dollar Roundtable, Independent Retired Football Players Summit, and the Supreme Courts of Delaware, Ohio, and Wyoming. Dr. Amen has been featured in *Newsweek*, *Parade*, *The New York Times Magazine*, *Men's Health,* and *Cosmopolitan*.

Dr. Amen is married, the father of four children, a grandfather, and an avid table tennis player.

Larry Momaya, M.D.

Larry Momaya, M.D. is a board-certified psychiatrist and is certified as a Master Practitioner of Hypnotherapy, NLP, and Time Empowerment Techniques®, including a powerful method called Time Line Therapy®, a process used to release the negative emotions of anger, sadness, fear, and guilt, as well as Limiting Decisions/Beliefs.

He takes an integrative approach in his work with people and uses a variety of techniques including hypnotherapy, visualization exercises, spirituality and meditation, music and sound, breathing techniques, practicing presence, several different psychotherapies, and a life-changing inquiry process called The Work of Byron Katie®.

Dr. Momaya enjoys working with people with emotional eating issues, mood and anxiety disorders, substance abuse problems, and ADHD, as well as spiritual, relationship, and self-esteem issues. He plays an integral role in educating the participants in the Amen Clinics weight-loss groups.

He has a keen interest in helping people shift their focus from the place of mental "dis-Ease" to moving towards mental wellness and personal empowerment. He founded a weekly experiential/educational group called The Path of Wellness (www.thepathofwellness.net) in early 2009, helping people come closer to finding their own inner peace through these various techniques.

Dr. Momaya also has a variety of other passions, particularly in the creative arts and media. He hosted his own psychiatry call-in talk show called "A Look Inside," as well as a music program on public radio, which was broadcast worldwide. He has filled in for Dr. Amen on his National radio show "Change Your Brain, Change Your Life," and is a highly sought after speaker.

AMEN CLINICS, INC.

Amen Clinics, Inc. (ACI) was established in 1989 by Daniel G. Amen, M.D. They specialize in innovative diagnosis and treatment planning for a wide variety of behavioral, learning, emotional and cognitive, and weight problems for children, teenagers, and adults. ACI has an international reputation for evaluating brain-behavior problems, such as attention deficit disorder (ADD), depression, anxiety, school failure, brain trauma, obsessive-compulsive disorders, aggressiveness, marital conflict, cognitive decline, brain toxicity from drugs or alcohol, and obesity. Brain SPECT imaging is performed in the Clinics. ACI has the world's largest database of brain scans for behavioral problems.

ACI welcomes referrals from physicians, psychologists, social workers, marriage and family therapists, drug and alcohol counselors, and individual clients.

Amen Clinics, Inc., Newport Beach
4019 Westerly Place, Suite 100
Newport Beach, CA 92660
(949) 266-3700

Amen Clinics, Inc., Fairfield
350 Chadbourne Road
Fairfield, CA 94585
(707) 429-7181

Amen Clinics, Inc., Northwest
616 120th Avenue, NE, Suite C100
Bellevue, WA 98005
(888) 564-2700, Ext. 4

Amen Clinics, Inc., DC
1875 Campus Commons Drive
Reston, VA 20191
(703) 860-5600
www.amenclinic.com

AMENCLINIC.COM

Amenclinic.com is an educational interactive brain website geared toward mental health and medical professionals, educators, students, and the general public. It contains a wealth of information to help you learn about our clinics and the brain. The site contains more than three hundred color brain SPECT images, thousands of scientific abstracts on brain SPECT imaging for psychiatry, BMI and calorie calculators, and much, much more.

View hundreds of astonishing color 3-D brain SPECT images on:
Aggression
Attention deficit disorder, including the six subtypes
Dementia and cognitive decline
Drug abuse
PMS
Anxiety disorders
Brain trauma
Depression
Obsessive-compulsive disorder
Stroke
Seizures